Neurodiversity: A Very Short Introduction

Very Short Introductions available now:

Available soon:

For more information visit our website

www.oup.com/vsi/

Robert Chapman
Sue Fletcher-Watson

NEURODIVERSITY

A Very Short Introduction

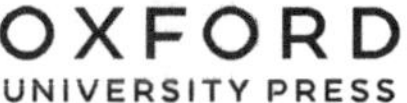

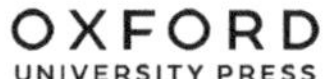

Great Clarendon Street, Oxford, OX2 6DP,
United Kingdom

Oxford University Press is a department of the University of Oxford.
It furthers the University's objective of excellence in research, scholarship,
and education by publishing worldwide. Oxford is a registered trade mark of
Oxford University Press in the UK and in certain other countries.

Published in the United States of America by Oxford University Press
198 Madison Avenue, New York, NY 10016, United States of America

British Library Cataloguing in Publication Data
Data available

Library of Congress Control Number: 2025938821

ISBN 9780198876519

DOI: 10.1093/9780191987915.001.0001

Printed and bound by
CPI Group (UK) Ltd., Croydon, CR0 4YY

The manufacturer's authorised representative in the EU for product safety is
Oxford University Press España S.A. of Parque Empresarial San Fernando de Henares,
Avenida de Castilla, 2 – 28830 Madrid (www.oup.es/en or product.safety@oup.com).
OUP España S.A. also acts as importer into Spain of products made by the manufacturer.

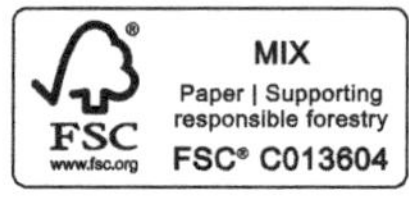

Preface

This book is about neurodiversity. Neurodiversity is a relatively new term, being coined in the 1990s by a community of autistic activists. Part of their idea was that, just as the ecosystem is enriched by biodiversity, so too is human society enriched by a diversity of ways of thinking. And just as biodiversity requires our collective effort to support and conserve, so too does neurodiversity. Based on this, these activists began to work towards a new civil rights and justice movement led by people with social and communication disabilities. They hoped this movement would advocate for social and legal reforms for autistic people as well as others whose sensory, cognitive, or neurological profiles set them apart from the norm.

Since these early days, the movement has grown rapidly. Now it includes not just autistic people, but people with all kinds of disabilities and divergences around the globe. Neurodiversity advocates include people who identify as anything from bipolar to dyspraxic and everything in between. We can describe them as neurodivergent. As such, there is now a large and still-growing movement of loosely connected individuals and groups usually known simply as the neurodiversity movement. This movement precisely seeks to change the world in the kinds of ways those early advocates specified.

The autistic scholar Nick Walker distinguished the neurodiversity movement from the emerging neurodiversity paradigm. This refers to the underlying assumptions or principles contingent upon neurodiversity's existence that represent a change in thinking, theory, and research necessary for the future that proponents of the movement have been collectively building. The point of this paradigm, for Walker, is to move away from framing minds or brains as either 'normal' or 'abnormal', and instead to begin with an embrace of neurological diversity as itself normal. For Walker, this shift will be relevant both for scientific research and for cultural representation of neurological variations. It will help move away from the prevalent assumption that neurodivergent people are necessarily broken or deficient, and towards a more inclusive framework for understanding, researching, and supporting mental variation.

From this view, a key point is that disablement is seen as related to politics and power rather than being a natural fact determined by individual ability alone. For instance, dyslexia is a disability largely because written text has become such a pivotal source of information and mode of communication. Similarly, insofar as autism is a matter of sensory-processing differences, the extent to which an autistic person is disabled will be determined by sensory environments such as the lights we use, sound levels, and so forth. This is an important insight since, if accepted, it has significant implications for how we should design schools, workplaces, and so forth. As such the neurodiversity movement seeks to challenge not just how we think about and study neurological variations, but also how we organize society in a variety of ways.

This book aims to introduce and synthesize a range of key themes in the theory, history, politics, and practice of neurodiversity. Here we describe, in simple terms, the history of the movement and its key innovations, concepts, controversies, and debates. This then allows us to cover the significance of the movement for politics, policy, and practice. In turn, this should help readers gain a basic understanding of what neurodiversity is all about, and then to decide what they want to explore further.

It is important to say up front that we recognize that there are different neurodiversity stakeholders and have worked to build this into our writing. We have written this book with at least three key groups in mind. First and foremost, we have written it for neurodivergent people, as well as their friends and families. To be clear, this is not a self-help book nor one which gives practical advice. Rather, it is meant to introduce readers to a new way of thinking about things usually called mental or neurodevelopmental 'disorders' and to help people navigate the various positions and debates within the neurodiversity movement. It also helps us think critically about concepts such as 'intelligence', 'ability', 'illness', and associated notions in new ways, and how these relate to forms of political domination. While we do not offer practical advice, we therefore hope this book will be valuable for developing a deeper understanding of self, others, and society. This in turn can be empowering through informing understanding of challenges that arise in day-to-day life as well as wider social and political issues.

Second, we have also written this book with researchers and practitioners in mind. We recognize that many people who study neurodivergence or work with neurodivergent people want to learn about the neurodiversity approach. However, most are trained in a more traditional medicalized approach grounded in the normalcy paradigm (a term indicating the currently dominant, medicalized approach, which we explain below). Moreover, they may not be able to find adequate resources for learning to update their understanding or may be met with conflicting advice or information where they find it. Of greatest concern is the large volume of misinformation we cover later in the section in Chapter 5 on *Neurodiversity-lite*. By providing an overview and synthesis of the theories and implications of the neurodiversity paradigm, we hope this book will be useful for researchers and professionals who wish to update their practice to incorporate the insights of the neurodiversity paradigm and support the goals of the neurodiversity movement.

Third, we have written this with students in mind. Neurodiversity theory is relevant to a wide range of fields, from sociology to psychology, education to philosophy. As such it is increasingly being brought into a range of both academic and vocational university courses. We have written this book in part to be useful to students who are seeking clarity on the neurodiversity approach. While our book is, we stress, a short introduction and therefore not comprehensive, we have developed it as a basis for further study.

Who are we?

Given our subject matter, we think it is important to be open about who we are and what each of us brings as well as the limitations of our knowledge and understanding. We are two academics from the UK who have both worked on neurodiversity theory and research for some time.

One author, Robert Chapman (they/them), is Assistant Professor in Critical Neurodiversity Studies at Durham University. They are autistic and also have first-hand experience of other neurodivergent disabilities and mental health conditions. They are white, nonbinary, and come from a working-class background and the foster care system. They began blogging on neurodiversity in the early 2010s while studying philosophy, before carrying out doctoral research on ethical issues relating to autism and neurodiversity between 2013 and 2018. Since then, they have remained active in various political campaigns and have published widely on neurodiversity theory and practice, as exemplified by their previous book *Empire of Normality: Neurodiversity and Capitalism*. As such, they bring an insider's perspective combined with a deal of relevant knowledge and expertise.

The second author, Sue Fletcher-Watson (she/her), is a Professor of Developmental Psychology at the University of Edinburgh. Sue identifies as neurotypical, while recognizing the limitations of this category—and any descriptor categories under the umbrella of neurodiversity. She has no personal experience of neurodivergence or mental ill-health. Sue is white, cisgender, pansexual, and came from a privileged background in terms of social class. Her immediate family is neurodiverse. Sue began consciously considering the neurodiversity paradigm in her work from about 2012 and then blogging and writing about neurodiversity more explicitly a few years later. Sue tries to apply the principles of the neurodiversity paradigm in her research and to produce evidence which can support neurodiversity-informed change in services. She does so in her own research projects by establishing partnerships with neurodivergent academics and mentoring neurodivergent students and by using participatory methods to link with neurodivergent people outside academia. Her expertise in participatory methods has resulted in highly cited key papers and awards. Sue attempts to use her leadership roles, for example as Editor-in-Chief of the journal *Autism* and as Director of the Salvesen Mindroom Research Centre at the University of Edinburgh, as a platform to raise the profile of the neurodiversity paradigm and embed its principles in academic work.

While we believe that our combined expertise and knowledge makes us well placed to write this introductory book, it is important to recognize that our knowledge is limited by our positionality and as such is far from perfect. As two white academics, born and based in the UK, our experiences are less relevant to members of racialized minorities and many people from the majority world. With this in mind, we have sought to emphasize throughout how important it is to recognize how race, ethnicity, culture, and neurodivergence intersect, and how this takes place within a global system that privileges white people at the expense of Black, Asian, Brown, and Indigenous peoples. Neurodiversity as a paradigm is largely grounded in Westernized models of thinking and there are alternative conceptual frameworks and traditions from around the globe which have not gained the same level of international currency and which we are not qualified to introduce with authority. Wherever possible, we instead signpost original scholarship for the reader to explore.

We are also aware that while neurodivergence is often associated with autism, it encompasses a wide range of diagnoses or disabilities. Nobody has direct experience of all of these, and we only have (direct and indirect) experience of a handful between us. As such, while much of this book draws on the work of autistic pioneers in neurodiversity activism and theory, we have sought to emphasize the relevance of neurodiversity to those with different experiences of mental disablement or distress, not just autistics. As we will come back to, we advocate for a broad, inclusive conception of neurodivergence.

More generally, we seek to follow what Black feminist author Kimberlé Crenshaw describes as an intersectional perspective. This emphasizes how people who sit at intersecting axes of oppression—say, people who are both Black and female, or neurodivergent and trans, and so on—often face more specific and complicated forms of oppression than those who are in one oppressed group, and which may be missed by efforts that focus on single group issues. By the same token, we frame neurodivergent liberation as bound up with collective liberation, and thus as part of a broader struggle for the freedoms of oppressed peoples globally. The power dynamics of neurodivergence sit within a broader system that bell hooks described as 'imperialist white-supremacist capitalist patriarchy'. We hope to make this clear as we guide readers through the various issues we cover.

Contents

Chapter 1
Introducing neurodiversity

A brief history of the movement

To understand the neurodiversity movement it will help to begin
with its history. For this we need to turn back to the early 1990s,
when autistic people first began gaining recognition for their
self-advocacy work. At this time autism was generally seen as a
terrible individual tragedy, and most researchers hoped to develop
a 'treatment' or 'cure' for autism. Autism itself was mainly defined
as a cognitive deficit in social understanding with biological
underpinnings. The thought was that new biomedical,
psychological, or behavioural intervention might help eliminate
this deficit. Most autism advocacy was dominated by the parents
of autistic children as well as concerned doctors. They mainly
adopted this dominant way of thinking about autism and thus
argued for greater funding for medical intervention and support.

This began to be challenged when autistic people were first able to
connect with each other online. This happened as the internet and
personal computers became more widely available in the early
1990s. Autism Network International, a pioneering effort run by
and for autistic people, was formed in 1992. In turn, some
tech-savvy autistics began making email lists and then chat rooms
for autistic people to discuss autism. The first was Autism
Network International's list from 1994. As more autistic people

gained access to the internet, and more were being diagnosed due to the broadening of the autism concept, many of them realized they found online communication much easier than in-person communication. Many also found that communicating with other autistics came more naturally to them than communicating with non-autistics.

Based on these experiences, early autistic self-advocates in an autistic-led email list called Independent Living (which was abbreviated to InLv)—a term taken from the earlier disability rights movement, emphasizing the importance of freeing disabled people from institutions—began arguing that many of the problems autistic people face were more about societal expectations and barriers rather than being intrinsic to autism. They also began suggesting that autistic people might have characteristic yet overlooked cognitive strengths, such as logical thinking or attention to detail. This sought to provide a more balanced view of autism that would reduce stigma and increase opportunity for autistic people. In the same years, the term 'neurotypical' began to be used—for instance on the satirical website by Laura Tisoncik, *The Institute for the Neurologically Typical*, which was a spoof of a medical institute that playfully reversed the medical gaze back on to those considered 'normal'. But the term also had a less humorous role, as online advocates were also talking about 'neurotypical' as just one of many equally legitimate ways of being, challenging the widespread assumption that it was the only correct way for a brain to be wired.

These new concepts, and the new politics surrounding them, were brought out of these groups by a journalist called Harvey Blume who wrote several articles in the late 1990s, including one in the *New York Times*, and then an *Atlantic* article that introduced the term 'neurodiversity' to a broader audience. Shortly after this, a then sociology student called Judy Singer used the word neurodiversity in a book chapter. This is the first known use in an academic source, though it is now considered inaccurate to credit

any single person with coining the word or birthing the idea.
Following these early publications, the movement grew rapidly,
and its theories were continually developed by an ever-growing
number of neurodivergent people. This was not just autistic
people, but also those with a wide range of other diagnoses, or
even with no official diagnosis at all. In time, groups such as the
Autistic Self-Advocacy Network, driven by advocates such as Ari
Ne'eman, began to exert significant political influence in the USA,
while the UK Labour Party would eventually develop a
'neurodiversity manifesto' led by neurodivergent members, and in
Chile a recently proposed new constitution included an explicit
commitment to neurodivergent liberation. The book *Neurotribes*
by the late Steve Silberman did a huge amount to bring
neurodiversity—and the autistic experience specifically—into the
mainstream. At the same time, grassroots and mutual aid
organizations such as the Autistic Women and Nonbinary
Network and the neurodivergent abolitionist organization
Neuromancers have been doing vital community organizing. All
this was able to happen because so many neurodivergent people
have organized together not just to fight for rights and justice,
but also to collectively develop the theories that we seek to
explain—and contribute to—in this book.

Defining neurodiversity

In this book we want to emphasize—following the work of a range
of neurodiversity activists and scholars—how useful it is to see
neurodiversity as bringing the possibility of a new scientific and
cultural *paradigm*. That is, we want to emphasize that it has the
potential to bring a mass shift in the fundamental way we think
about, study, and respond to people across the whole neurological
spectrum of humanity. Part of what we want to establish is that
this could help improve our scientific understanding and
professional practice alongside understandings of politics and
culture. At the same time, we want to show how this has radical
potential to be liberating for people with a wide range of

disabilities, and ultimately helpful for everyone, including neurotypicals. This is because it will help us change how we carry out research, approach clinical practice, and think about policy and law, among other things.

In this chapter we will explain this in more detail. Our framing of the neurodiversity paradigm emphasizes two core principles: affirm complexity and politicize neuronormativity. Together these principles capture the applied consequences of neurodiversity. Application of these principles will constitute a paradigm shift. As such, we will begin by saying a bit more about what the words 'paradigm' and 'paradigm shift' mean and why they are important. We then provide a brief history of the neurodiversity movement and clarify some of the key concepts of its proponents. This will put us in a good place to return to our two key principles and our definition of the neurodiversity paradigm as we understand it.

What is a scientific paradigm?

A scientific paradigm, at base, is a set of assumptions, principles, practices, and commitments that groups of researchers or practitioners share to get their work done, for a given historical period. Looked at this way, every science has a dominant paradigm at any given time, which can then change as our understanding progresses. For instance, in physics we might talk of Newton's paradigm and Einstein's paradigm, since each of these pioneering thinkers in turn established different fundamental theories that the scientists who followed them then relied on to do their own research. Or in biology we might talk of there being different paradigms before and after Darwin's theory of evolution became widely accepted by other biologists.

A paradigm shift occurs whenever a new theoretical framework comes along that radically changes how research and scholarship in a given field operates. Every now and again, as the dominant

paradigm of a given field becomes outdated or struggles to
accommodate new data, new approaches with different
assumptions and theoretical bases are proposed. Ideally, one of
these will become widely adopted to guide scientists working in
the respective field—if not, the field might split into factions
adopting different paradigms. Paradigm shifts should improve
the work of scientists by better explaining recent findings and
opening up new lines of enquiry.

Consider another clear example of such a shift: the Copernican
revolution in cosmology. Shifting from viewing the earth at the
centre of the solar system to viewing the sun at the centre of the
solar system changed some of the most fundamental assumptions
that cosmologists were working with, allowing them to develop a
vastly improved scientific understanding of the cosmos. More
generally, then, when we look at the development of science in this
way, we might say that all our mature sciences have paradigms,
and that paradigms are temporary (albeit sometimes long-lasting)
frameworks shared by the majority of those in the given field. And
we can add that, in time, our current paradigms will no doubt be
replaced by future ones as our scientific understanding continues
to develop.

Of course, our sciences are not totally separate from each other,
and often paradigms overlap or are shared between different
fields. When it comes to scientific understandings of
neurodiversity, we are concerned with a range of disciplines and
fields. Important here are both the 'psych' sciences and fields,
which includes psychiatry, psychology, psychometrics, as well as
the 'neuro' sciences, such as neurology or neuro-psychology. In
turn, we are also concerned with how these relate to biology and
genetics, which are often deployed in efforts to explain variations
in cognitive and emotional functioning. We are equally concerned
with more applied and social science approaches relating to
therapy, education, and so forth. We are concerned with all of
these as, together, they are the cluster of sciences that are used to

determine policy and practice when it comes to human neurodiversity—both neurotypicals and neurodivergents.

What about cultural paradigm shifts?

We can also talk about shifts in cultural paradigms. This would refer to similarly fundamental shifts regarding how we understand aspects of human diversity, arts, cultural practices, and so on. They may also relate to social attitudes, norms, and practices. Consider the shift from seeing homosexuality as a mental illness in the 20th century to seeing being gay, lesbian, or queer as minority sexual orientations related to our own cultural practices and histories, of which we can be proud. We might say that this, alongside feminism, helped propel—although did not complete, since many queer people still face all kinds of stigma and discrimination—a mass cultural paradigm shift relating to sexual and gendered norms. This cultural shift is why, for instance in the UK, like some other countries, gay marriage is now legal, and LGBTQ pride events now happen all over the nation.

Importantly, this progress has been made in significant part through the campaigning of a great many LGBTQ activists and organizers, who put in decades of hard work with many risks to push for mass cultural change. This includes artists, writers, and so on who have played important roles in creating the space to celebrate LGBTQ cultures. Similarly to this, along with the attempt to develop a scientific paradigm shift, neurodivergent activists, artists, writers, creators, and organizers have, over recent decades, begun the significant project of starting a paradigm shift in cultural understandings, norms, and practices relating to neurodiversity. Many neurodivergent artists now create explicitly neurodivergent arts, and it is becoming more common for neurodivergent characters to be portrayed in humane and inclusive ways in literature and film. As we will see, the attempt at developing a paradigm shift is also highly relevant for research in the arts and humanities, including disability theory, which is no less important, and perhaps more fundamental, for the neurodiversity movement than the attempt at a paradigm shift in the sciences. Neurodiversity theory can help us rethink our histories, the significance of neurodivergent art, and much else.

The normalcy paradigm

The term we use for the currently dominant paradigm for studying and responding to neurodiversity is the normalcy paradigm. Nick Walker, a leading thinker and scholar in the neurodiversity movement, called this 'the pathology paradigm'. While we broadly follow Walker's analysis, we use the term normalcy paradigm rather than her preferred term pathology paradigm. We call it this because the core issue is not the recognition of mental or neurological pathology as such, but rather the conflation of normalcy and health, and thus atypicality with pathology. Overcoming the normalcy paradigm is not about rejecting the very concept of mental or neurological pathology, variations of which are ancient and can be found across different cultures globally. Rather, it is about overcoming the *default* pathologization of people or groups who are atypical and thereby at risk of struggling. The neurodiversity paradigm recognizes and empowers all people who fall outside neuronormativity, regardless of health or disability status.

Importantly, neurodiversity proponents take the normalcy paradigm to be dominant both in culture and in scientific understandings, not least since science is, after all, a human cultural practice, aiming at objectivity while intimately intertwined with all sorts of cultural normative assumptions. Indeed, for neurodiversity proponents, it is important to try to shift both cultural and scientific paradigms simultaneously, since the assumptions of each are intertwined with and enforce those of the other.

To briefly consider another parallel in historic social justice movements, we can compare what neurodiversity activists are trying to achieve with the past achievements of anti-racist movements. While the work needed to combat both interpersonal and institutional racism is barely started, shifts have been made that shape both cultural and scientific understandings. Importantly, the modern understanding of race as a social construction (which is not diminished in its impact by that understanding) has come from a combination of activism, creative artefacts (e.g. literature, theatre, fine arts), scholarship in the arts and humanities, and scientific discovery.

The dominant paradigm is most centrally defined by assuming a relatively restricted *normal* range when it comes to mental or neurological functioning. Within this approach, it is further assumed that if someone falls outside this norm and is struggling in any way then there must be something wrong with them. That is, it is thought that some part of their brain or mind is broken and in need of fixing. We see this, for instance, in the use of the psychiatric word 'disorder', as in developmental language disorder (DLD) or attention deficit hyperactivity disorder (ADHD). The term indicates a problem stemming from an underlying dysfunction. Similarly, in neuroscientific research on neurodivergent people, differences in brain structure or functioning are routinely interpreted as deficits, when a value-neutral interpretation would be more reasonable, given our still minimal comprehension of how the brain actually works. Indeed, even the distinctive abilities and positive qualities of neurodivergent people can be pathologized, as in a 1991 journal article describing an 'autism-specific deception impairment'. We also see this restricted normal range in the scientific search to find 'cures' or 'treatments' for such disabilities, at biological and psychological levels. In therapies, many likewise seek to erase 'abnormal' behaviours or thoughts and to promote 'normal' ones. What unites each of these is the assumption of a restricted normal range, and the further assumption that it is bad to fall outside the normal range. This why we say these sciences share a general normalcy paradigm.

Relatedly, especially in modern capitalist societies we also see a broader cultural normalcy paradigm, whereby neurodivergence is often automatically seen to be a tragic deviation or something to be ashamed of in society more generally. Following a diagnosis, whether of Down syndrome or dyscalculia (aka developmental coordination disorder, or DCD), parents often feel a sense of grief on finding that their child is not 'normal'. We also see such assumptions manifesting when children are bullied for being 'weird' or adults are feared for being 'crazy'. These patterns are reinforced by representations on film which frequently use the atypical behaviour of neurodivergent characters to produce dramatic events to drive the plot forward—as in the film *Rain Man*, when the character of Raymond Babbitt has a meltdown in an airport, forcing his brother to drive him across the USA. Both in our sciences and in our broader culture, then, it is widely assumed that normal is good and abnormal is bad. This is what neurodiversity proponents mean when they say the normalcy paradigm is the *dominant* paradigm. To say that it is dominant is to say that it underlies and structures the standard ways we think about, study, represent, and respond to variations in cognitive or emotional functioning. Black neurodivergent scholars Chantelle Jessica Lewis and Jason Arday have referred to this cultural dominance as 'neurotypical hegemony', indicating how it closes off other ways of understanding and relating to ourselves, each other, and the world around us.

While much of the way neurodivergent and neurotypical people are understood is often just seen as established fact, it may surprise some readers to be told that the idea of the 'normal' person is relatively recent. Prior to the 19th century, health and illness were usually seen as a matter of balance and imbalance rather than being associated with normality and abnormality. To any doctor working in the year 1800, the idea of a 'normal' person or of a 'normal' heart rate, lung capacity, intelligence, and so forth would not make much sense. In fact, while much more abstract conceptions of the average date back to Pythagoras in ancient Greece, their use for conceptualizing concrete things only began when astronomers first developed concepts of normality to track stars in the early 19th century.

It was following this, in the 1830s, that the notion of the average began to be applied to people and populations. In 1835 the Belgian social scientist Adolphe Quetelet proposed the notion of the 'average man' for the first time, based on comparing measurements of soldiers and then working out their average height, weight, and so forth. This fitted with a modern capitalist and swiftly industrializing society that required humans to adjust to standardized machinery in the workplace, and which valued people in relation to their purported individual productive capacities. It changed how we thought about, studied, and responded to illness and disability in a very significant way. It was in this context that the normalcy paradigm began to be developed. Scientists such as Francis Galton drew on Quetelet to propose that human mental functioning could be ranked in relation to a 'normal' range. Importantly, Galton was also a white supremacist who wrote books seeking to rank the races in terms of cognitive ability. While his more overt racism is now widely rejected, his underlying framework nonetheless came to underpin much thinking in the psychological and neuro-sciences since this time, not to mention shifting broader cultural understandings that position people as subnormal (disabled), normal (abled), or supernormal (gifted) in terms of their bodily or mental functioning. From this time on, much of our science has assumed that we can rank all aspects of mental or bodily functioning in relation to a normal range, and moreover that we should try to make people more normal if they fall outside that range.

Another scientific tradition which has shaped our concept of 'normal' is the history of neuropsychology, grounded in adult case studies. Before brain imaging techniques became widespread, the only insight into the functions of different brain regions came from cases where 'normal' brain function had been grossly disrupted, often by injury or stroke. The famous case of Phineas Gage, a railway worker who survived a massive injury to his frontal lobes at work, provided much of the early understanding of that brain region's role in what we now term 'executive functions'. This focus on people who had abilities that were lost as a result of injury reinforces the direct correspondence between atypical and unhealthy. More than just this, a simplistic mapping of specific brain regions to cognitive, emotional, or sensorimotor functions generated a modular notion of the brain and shaped a largely fruitless and expensive quest to identify regional anomalies in the brain associated with specific diagnoses.

Sometimes, of course, concepts of 'normality' have been very useful. When it comes to relatively simple organs, such as the heart, a sense of the 'normal' heart rate has for the most part been useful for understanding when we should be worried about any given person's health, and what a healthy range might look like. But in other cases, this approach has been far more controversial. Often the norms we construct have a racialized or gendered bias due to studies only focusing on certain parts of the population. This can lead to biased results that impact access to healthcare for marginalized people. Even in the seemingly simple example of a 'normal' heart rate, reliance on data drawn from a limited population (in terms of gender or race) produces unhelpfully narrow or skewed expectations. Similarly, our conceptions of 'normal' body weight may reinforce harmful and unrealistic pressures that all bodies should be the same specific kind of idealized body type.

Most relevantly for our purposes, the idea of the 'normal' brain or mind may contribute to stigma, misunderstanding, and support for harmful practices. In one trial, children with working memory problems were offered targeted training: the intervention improved working memory test scores, but did not generalize to better learning outcomes. In fact, these children ended up doing worse in their school maths tests, because they had missed maths lessons to do the working memory training. Neurodiversity proponents question whether we should retain the idea of an objectively 'normal' brain at all, if by 'normal' we mean correctly functioning. We now acknowledge that there is no correct sexuality, culture, or ethnicity, so why should we think there is a correct way for brains to develop? Likewise, we recognize that while a marginalized identity, such as being queer, may lead to societal disadvantage, the solution is not to change the person, but to change their circumstances. Neurodiversity proponents, and others, argue for the same approach to understanding and supporting neurodivergent people. When we consider these kinds of problems and questions, we can see that it might be time to develop a new paradigm. This would be one that doesn't discriminate based on an arbitrary standard of normality, let alone standards determined by the needs of the capitalist economy rather than those of humans.

The need for a neurodiversity paradigm

The neurodiversity movement is the movement of people who are advocating for liberation of neurodivergent people. While there are influential neurodiversity activists, the movement has no leader and is made up of loosely connected individuals and groups across the globe. Anyone who advocates for justice for neurodivergent people in the various ways we describe in this book might be said to be part of the movement.

This is where the idea of the neurodiversity paradigm comes in. Walker suggests that a key goal of the neurodiversity movement can be understood as a widespread supplanting of the normalcy paradigm with the neurodiversity paradigm. This is her term for the theoretical, scientific, and cultural paradigm Walker sees as being built by neurodiversity proponents. In particular, she associates this emerging paradigm with a rejection of the idea of the 'normal' brain or mind being associated with the average range. Instead, it begins with an embrace of neurological diversity as itself 'normal' or natural. Here Walker follows earlier advocates, such as those on Independent Living, Harvey Blume, and Judy Singer, who suggest that just in the way it is 'normal' for a forest or meadow to have a diverse ecosystem, so too is it 'normal' for humanity to have a diversity of kinds of minds.

In this view, the fact that we discriminate against some minds and not others does not reflect a natural order, but rather current societal value. Consider the case of left-handedness, which was discriminated against historically. There is nothing inherently wrong with being left-handed, despite it being statistically rare, yet in the past left-handed people were forced to learn to use their right hands, rather than to embrace their natural disposition to use their left hands. While left-handedness is thought to be underpinned by neurological differences, and is atypical, we can now clearly see that left-handed people were not disordered and in need of fixing. Rather, they were punished because they were socially marginalized. The attempt to shift from the normalcy paradigm to a still emerging neurodiversity paradigm is partially analogous to this shift in understandings of handedness. After all, scientists still study left-handedness, and it is still acknowledged in educational settings, but without the unduly negative framing that was previously so widespread.

As to the political significance of this shift, let us consider a second partial analogy. The attempt to build a neurodiversity paradigm follows a similar pattern of change we have already begun to see when it comes to other kinds of ethnic and cultural diversity. In the 19th century, for instance, many white British people, including leading scientists, thought that there was a natural hierarchy of races, with white people at the top. But now we know that was grounded in a racist worldview, and that no ethnicity is better than any other. Importantly, this shift is not just attitudinal—a progressive reframing in response to social pressure—but genuinely paradigmatic. We now believe the concept of race is socially constructed and has no basis in genetics, nor biology more generally. Moreover, we recognize that 19th-century attempts to rank the races scientifically were infused with white supremacist ideological and cultural baggage. These previous scientists thought that their view was objective, but we have since switched our paradigm. Scientists now study ethnic diversity among humans in a very different way, usually not grounded in a racist worldview to anything like the same extent. We say 'to the same extent' because racism does still affect scientific research to some degree, but it seems clear that there has been some progress in both scientific and cultural understandings since the 19th century.

It is important to note here that our current way of ranking brains and minds grew together, historically, with these earlier attempts to rank by race. Often it was the same scientists, such as Francis Galton, developing both sets of ranking. This relates to how racism was built into the origins of both capitalism and modern imperialism, as Black studies scholars such as Cedric Robinson have detailed. As with the study of ethnic diversity, making a shift away from these views when it comes to human neurological variation should similarly lead to a totally different way of conceptualizing, researching, and responding to issues relating to human neurodiversity. Following this partial analogy, we can see that the attempt to build a new paradigm is not just about improving scientific research, but also about cultivating disability justice and neurodivergent liberation. If we can build a better paradigm, the shift may in turn help us see how to build a better world that is more inclusive of neurodivergent people. The potential is not just for an improvement in scientific understanding, but also for moral progress, and to reorganize our society in a way that is liberating for everyone who falls outside the overly restrictive boundaries of the normalcy paradigm. This is an important part of what we want to establish throughout this book.

Contested and evolving terminology

Before we clarify how we understand the neurodiversity paradigm, it is important to consider that the neurodiversity paradigm comes with a new set of terms and concepts. Yet we should also caveat that, as with all words and concepts, their meanings change over time, and which are most useful will continue to change. Doubtless readers of the future will reject some of the language we use, as thinking and discourse moves forward. Even at this moment in time, there is no single set of words that are necessarily associated with the neurodiversity paradigm or which all neurodiversity proponents use in the precise same way. And even those that are more often associated with it can be challenged or reinterpreted. Moreover, throughout this book we will draw parallels between the neurodiversity movement and other liberation movements and attempt to explore the intersectionality of those movements. The terminology of those communities is likewise shifting and evolving, and so it is certain that language we use here will be replaced over time.

Still, in recent decades, at least a fairly coherent set of important terms and concepts has emerged, which we will adopt in this book. It will help to give some definitions before we go any further.

By 'neuro' we are primarily referring to things to do with the brain or nervous system. This in turn is intimately intertwined with our mental life and our cognitive and emotional functioning. Often, when we say 'neuro' we will make the reasonable assumption that there is a link between neurological processes (e.g. synaptic firing, blood-flow in the brain) and mental processes—those relating to cognition or emotion—even if we don't know exactly how this works yet in any given case. At the same time, though, we also make the equally reasonable and important assumption that mental functioning cannot be reduced to neurology. This is because mental functioning is also determined by all sorts of other things. These include other parts of the body, our social learning and relationships with other people, our current environment, our past experiences, our culture, and much else. Thus, when we say 'neuro' we mean it in a purposely broad sense, acknowledging how complex are the interactions between brain, body, and world that together constitute each of our mental lives.

'Diversity' indicates that there is variation, and is a trait that only groups can have, not individuals. Combined with 'neuro', 'neurodiversity' refers to variations in neurological and nervous system functioning that we can say any given group has to a greater or lesser extent. For instance, a group of four people where one is autistic, another dyspraxic, another with ADHD, and another with schizophrenia would be a relatively neurologically diverse group. By contrast, a group of four where everyone has the same diagnosis, or where nobody qualifies for any diagnosis, would likely be relatively neurologically uniform. Importantly, it would not make sense to call an individual 'neurodiverse' unless they literally had multiple brains that were different from each other. For the most part, only groups can be neurodiverse, not individuals.

The next important term is 'neurotypical'. This is a term developed by neurodiversity proponents to refer to people who are considered to function 'normally', and thus who do not qualify for diagnoses of neurological disabilities. A neurotypical person might otherwise be described as 'typically developed' or as falling within the 'normal range' of cognitive and emotional functioning. It is important to emphasize, however, that in the neurodiversity paradigm this is not taken to refer to a natural grouping of people. Rather, who is considered normal will be determined by social norms of a given society. This in turn will be determined by the economic system, the state of technology, religious and ideological beliefs, and many other factors. Put another way, 'neurotypicals' refers to a rough cluster of people who sit in a fairly central place within the neurological power structures of a given society or global system. To recognize them as neurotypicals is to recognize their socially privileged position, rather than suggesting they are normal in a more objective sense, such as having a shared, identifiable essence in their brains.

In contrast to the neurotypical are those who are neurodivergent (coined by Kasianne Asasumasu). Just as neurotypical refers to anyone who falls closer to the normative ideal of the society, those who are neurodivergent fall outside that ideal. There is no strict or clear dividing line since these norms themselves have some level of vagueness and also shift. But neurodivergence is generally associated with people who struggle to function in line with the neurological norms of a society, whose needs are less commonly met within standard systems (e.g. mainstream school classrooms), and who are discriminated against specifically in light of this. Some people might choose to identify as multiply neurodivergent where they have more than one overlapping profile that would on its own be considered neurodivergent—for example, people with a diagnosis of ADHD and autism. However, the term neurodivergent is not meant to be limited to those with one of a specific list of diagnoses, and so identifying as neurodivergent alone can capture any profile outside the current norm. Individuals who are neurodivergent might also use other language to describe themselves, such as neuro-atypical, or a specific diagnostic label, such as dyspraxic. Of course, every individual can and should use terminology they prefer, and in this book we are more concerned with language we can use when talking in general terms about neurodiversity.

Most neurodivergent people are disabled, although there are also neurodivergent people who are only marginally neurodivergent, not to the point of being disabled. For instance, left-handedness can be seen as a form of marginal neurodivergence. While left-handed people are no longer stigmatized, many things, from scissors to guitars, are still typically built for right-handed people, and this can sometimes be a problem for those who are left-handed. We also include degenerative illnesses such as dementia, mental health conditions such as bipolar disorder or schizophrenia, and some neurologically based physical conditions, such as epilepsy, in neurodivergence. Neurodivergence can be non-medical (as in the case of left-handedness) or medical (as in the case of epilepsy). Thus while 'neurodivergence' helps us talk about minds that fall outside the 'norm' without pathologizing them, this term alone does not imply any particular health status. This is important to remember because, even though the neurodiversity movement exists partly to move away from default pathologization, people with disorders also face systemic forms of injustice and human rights abuses on account of diverging from neuronormativity, no less than wrongfully pathologized neurodivergent people.

A helpful term for groups of neurodivergent people is 'neurominority' (coined by Nick Walker). These are minority groups of people with at least vaguely similar traits in their cognitive or emotional functioning. Usually so far, this term has been used to reclaim psychiatric diagnoses such as autism or ADHD, and to reinterpret them in line with the neurodiversity paradigm framing. It is important to emphasize, however, that such classifications could have been different. They are as they are given complex historical circumstances rather than being natural groupings. For instance, 'autism' is a concept that has continually shifted since being termed in the early 20th century, as various social, economic, and political factors relating to sensory and emotional processing continue to change. There is also lots of overlap between many neurominorities and variation within any given one. Two autistic people might be very different from each other, while some autistic people are quite similar, cognitively speaking, to some people with ADHD. In this, neurominorities have some level of similarity with other kinds of minorities. Our conceptions of race and ethnicity, for instance, are not natural groupings, but rather reflect complex historical conditions that led to certain naming conventions for groups of people with roughly similar clusters of traits. Similarly, neurominorities are not natural groupings, but rather reflect the power structures of a given age, which lead us to notice some clusters of traits more than others.

Finally, 'neuronormativity' refers to societal valuations of different kinds of neurological or cognitive functioning. The term was developed in particular to challenge default assumptions that some kinds of brains or minds are just inherently superior or inferior to others: for instance, that neurotypicality is superior to neurodivergence. Instead of seeing our current societal cognitive hierarchies as timeless and objective, the concept of neuronormativity draws attention to how our neurological norms always reflect not just natural differences in functioning, but also contingent societal and cultural expectations.

There is also some language associated with the normalcy paradigm which is worth briefly defining, since neurodiversity is often making efforts to explain, interpret, and sometimes replace these categories. Most forms of neurodivergence, under the normalcy paradigm, would fall into one of five categories. Learning difficulties (also called specific learning difficulties) are those forms of neurodivergence most apparent in education contexts, and often diagnosed within the school system rather than by clinicians. Examples include dyslexia, dyscalculia, and dysgraphia. A learning disability, by contrast, is diagnosed in the presence of an IQ score below 70, representing a relatively comprehensive challenge to learning new information. Many individuals with a learning disability will also have some kind of genetic syndrome, such as Down syndrome, fragile x syndrome, or Williams syndrome, which commonly entails a low IQ test score along with other common features. A neurodevelopmental disorder (or condition) is normally diagnosed by a clinician, often a psychologist, and is a lifelong diagnosis which usually becomes apparent in childhood and shapes developmental pathways. Examples include ADHD, autism, and developmental language disorder. With the exception of stimulants for people with ADHD, it is rare for any of these three categories to be treated with medications—though many may take medicines for co-occurring difficulties like anxiety or poor sleep. A mental disorder or mental illness is usually diagnosed by a psychiatrist and often medications are a primary treatment option. Examples of things widely considered mental disorders include bipolar disorder, schizophrenia, and obsessive-compulsive disorder. Though many may be chronic, they are not necessarily considered lifelong and cures are both pursued and, in some cases, achieved. Finally, there is a range of neurodegenerative disorders including the dementias, Parkinson's disease, and motor neurone disease. These tend to arise in middle-to-late life and represent a degeneration in cognitive, affective, and sensorimotor abilities. One prominent form of neurodivergence that isn't neatly represented in these categories is epilepsy (and other seizure disorders). Any person falling into one or more of these groups might consider themselves disabled, depending on their context, experience, and identity. Of note, these definitions adhere to standard UK usage and may vary around the world—for example in the USA the term 'learning *disability*' can be used to refer to what we call 'learning *difficulties*', while Americans would use 'intellectual disability' for the UK's 'learning disability'. More broadly, outside of the terms developed in Western psychiatry over the last two centuries, there are countless further terms and concepts that name various forms of things we refer to as neurodivergence, relative to each culture and place. We advocate a version of the neurodiversity paradigm that holds space for a range of understandings from around the globe.

How we understand the neurodiversity paradigm

Now we have covered some—although by no means all—basic concepts and history, we are in a position to return to the understanding of the neurodiversity paradigm we adopt for this book. Before we get to this, it is important to emphasize that while there are more or less helpful ways to understand the neurodiversity paradigm, there is no single or correct way to conceptualize it. Especially since it is something that is still emerging and continually changing, any attempt to summarize it will remain incomplete.

Still, for the purposes of this book, one way of thinking about it is to break it down into core principles, which together fit well with the kinds of efforts we associate with the neurodiversity movement. While there are various valid ways to do this, for this book we suggest that in its simplest form, we can associate the neurodiversity paradigm with two core principles: affirm complexity and politicize neuronormativity. We will now explain these in turn, and how they differ from the normalcy paradigm, before going on to apply them throughout this book.

Affirm complexity

To explain what we mean by affirm complexity, it is first worth noting that all science is value-laden to at least some extent. This is because science is a human activity and everything humans do is driven by what our values are. We study chemistry, for instance, because we value understanding and manipulating the natural world, while we study medicine because we value health. That science is a value-laden activity is simply part of what science is, and thus is not, in itself, a bad thing. However, sometimes science and practice can at least implicitly be driven by ideological values that may end up being oppressive or harmful. This is part of the issue we identify in the normalcy paradigm and hope to correct with the alternative principles of the neurodiversity paradigm.

In our view, the normalcy paradigm is, in significant part, driven by the aim of controlling neurological complexity across the human population. Sometimes controlling biological heterogeneity is good. For instance, it is good for scientists to try to control cancer, diabetes, or dementia. But the normalcy paradigm takes the need to control heterogeneity too far. This paradigm is both based on, and reinforces, an overvaluation of cognitive and emotional uniformity and order in the human population. We can see this when we consider that much of our medical and psychological research and practice assumes that neurological heterogeneity is always a bad thing, and that neurological divergence is something we should always try to correct. The issue is that this seeks to control our species-level neurological heterogeneity in line with how we seek to control things like cancer or diabetes. This can be detrimental for people who are atypical but who do not want to be controlled, and indeed who find pressures to conform harmful.

We also see this overvaluation of uniformity manifesting in how diagnoses are conceived of. Consider the example of autism. As with many other diagnoses, much research on autism has been geared to finding an autistic 'essence' in the genes, brain, or cognition of autistic people. The implicit point of this is to be able to control autism, for instance by developing a prenatal test for terminating autistic foetuses or finding a neurological marker that could be used to identify autistic infants and shape their environment to 'prevent' them from 'becoming' autistic. So far, we have not found underlying biomarkers for autism, and within the normalcy paradigm this is seen as a failure. Indeed, in response to this perceived failure, some researchers suggest that the classification of autism lacks utility or should be abandoned in favour of more specific classifications that would map onto clear biomarkers. While individual researchers on this quest may not be seeking to control individual autistic people, the general endeavour serves to control in terms of being able to predict who is autistic and shape them into a more 'normal' ideal. Notably too, these kinds of efforts and discourses are not limited to autism, but are also something we see in many other similar diagnoses, from dyslexia to ADHD. As with autism, most learning difficulties and mental disorders have no known single biomarker, and often this leads to calls to abandon or refine such classifications. This looks more like people being adapted to serve science, rather than the opposite way around.

While normalcy paradigm science is surely genuine science—rather than pseudoscience—it is guided by implicit values for uniformity that undermine our ability to recognize, support, and value a wider range of human neurodiversity. By contrast, we suggest, the neurodiversity paradigm does not see uniformity (or even more precise classification) as the goal. For instance, when it comes to the autism classification, neurodiversity proponents tend to embrace the heterogeneity within the autistic population. They more often see this heterogeneity as part of what constitutes autistic community and culture. From the neurodiversity paradigm perspective, then, it is not necessarily a failure of our disability classifications that they contain diversity. Rather, it is a source of the richness of the communities that form around them. After all, a community or culture where everyone was identical would most likely lack the kind of richness that comes with including more diversity. Hence the neurodiversity perspective more often embraces heterogeneity at the level of the classification.

More broadly, from a neurodiversity approach, we should also affirm complexity at the species level. Rather than automatically seeing divergence from the norm as something to be feared or controlled, we should precisely expect divergence at the population level and should base our research, practice, and policy on this expectation. After all, it is not just that many of us are born diverging from the statistically normal neurological functioning. It is also that *all of us*, including neurotypicals, become neurodivergent if we live long enough. This can be through accidents that impact cognitive functioning, acquired impairments such as those associated with long Covid, or, ultimately, cognitive decline and degenerative diseases such as Alzheimer's in later life. Affirming complexity requires recognizing that there are a diverse range of support needs across the human spectrum, and that all should be accommodated regardless of how far from the norm they fall. It also requires having medical care in place for those conditions where this is relevant, such as epilepsy or dementia.

A related requirement of the demand to affirm complexity is to recognize the strength and opportunity that arises from our naturally occurring diversity. This is an important way to embed the call for recognition of the many and varied ways that individuals bring value to our society. The radical potential of the idea rests on recognition that heterogeneity in the human race—or in any subgroup of that whole—is in itself a source of strength and creativity.

On a practical level, for instance, diversity between people means we bring different experiences and views to the table and propose varied solutions to the challenges in our lives and society. This may have concrete benefits: diversity drives creativity and innovation as we spark ideas from each other and work collectively to tackle the many and varied barriers we each encounter in our lives. One study, for instance, found that adding one person with ADHD to a group of 'normal' controls made that group significantly better at creative problem solving, despite ADHD being associated with disability at the individual level. But more than this, a benefit of collective variety is the requirement to empathize—a society where everyone is the same is a society where we no longer need to imagine someone else's perspective or experience, nor work to escape our own narrow view.

To be clear, affirming complexity does not mean overlooking difficulties or never trying to control neurodivergent traits. For instance, we think it is vital to develop treatments to target diseases such as Alzheimer's, alongside socially supporting those with this condition. However, even in this relatively clear-cut example, an over-focus on the former and under-investment in the latter is a cause for concern. Our sole approach to neurodivergence—even in its most negative form—cannot be prevention and elimination. We must also incorporate support and understanding. Affirming complexity is about acknowledging that neurological diversity is inevitable and often forms part of the richness of human cultures as much as it is associated with illness or disability. Neurodiversity must shape our research, practice, and policy to accommodate that, so that neurodivergent people can thrive across the spectrum of humanity, regardless of whether we are healthy, disabled, or ill.

Politicize neuronormativity

The second principle is politicize neuronormativity. Neuronormativity regards how we evaluate which forms of neurological functioning are desirable or undesirable, and how this relates to what we consider normal or not. Often, the way we rank different kinds of minds is simply seen as natural. For instance, it is often assumed that having higher intelligence is simply naturally and objectively better than having lower intelligence. It is also often assumed that being 'normal' is simply inherently better than being disabled, and so on.

Politicizing neuronormativity challenges this through several interrelated commitments. Broadly, these question the way neurological or cognitive ability has often been constructed as an individual or natural matter. This is important, for us, as part of the power of the normalcy paradigm has precisely been to make things like autism or dyslexia seem like natural and individual dysfunctions rather than relationally constituted disabilities. Politicizing neuronormativity resists this naturalization, and helps us better understand the nature and working of neuronormativity.

The first way the paradigm commits to this is to always view what counts as 'normal' or 'healthy' neurological, cognitive, or behavioural functioning as itself something that occurs in a specific social and historical context. This is not to reject that the use of population averages can have scientific utility—as in the case of using a normal distribution of blood pressure to identify individuals whose blood pressure is worryingly low or high. Neither is it to deny that some conception of mental or neurological health or pathology is vital for medical science and healthcare as we know it. Rather, it is to acknowledge that while these often can have utility from a scientific and humanitarian perspective, they are nonetheless always mediated by cultural and economic norms. For instance, dyslexia only came to be seen as a pathology in literate societies that functioned through standardized schooling. In preliterate societies people we would now call dyslexic would have existed, but they would not have been disabled. Moreover, concepts of pathology always arise within and often reproduce unjust power relations of a given time and place. For example, women who resist patriarchal oppression have been pathologized as 'hysterical', when in fact they were responding to their oppression in a reasonable way. Similarly, Black civil rights activists in the USA in the 1960s were pathologized as having a 'protest psychosis'. Being aware of the political nature of neuronormativity, and how it relates not just to disability but also other intersections, is thus vital.

The second key way neuronormativity is politicized is in terms of how we understand ability and disability. In the normalcy paradigm, these have tended to be understood as individual attributes, which could either be stronger or weaker when compared to comparable attributes in other people. But the neurodiversity perspective, while acknowledging that individual biology is part of what grounds abilities, always sees them as socially, relationally, and collectively produced. That is, whether any given neurological or cognitive trait turns out to be useful or not will depend on a range of contextual factors. This includes what the task is, what technology or resources the individual has access to, the immediate environment they are in and how it was constructed, who they are working with, their motivation, and so forth.

Relatedly, it is also important to consider that whether people tend to count as 'strong' or 'weak' is also culturally produced. For example, whether we see a disposition to be highly emotional and cry in response to personal tragedy as strong or weak will depend on cultural norms, not to mention expectation relating to age, gender, race, and so forth. For instance, there is often more pressure on Black women to seem strong and to not cry, while white women may find they experience comparatively more support when they cry. This is important to note because, often, and at any given time, people will assume that their cultural norms relating to emotional and cognitive dispositions are objective, correct, or universal. But in fact they are contingent, and since cultural norms can be oppressive for those who fall outside them, finding ways to position our understandings of ability and disability in these ways is also a vital part of the neurodiversity paradigm lens.

Overall, acknowledging all of this and making all efforts to be vigilant of the potential ways neuronormativity can reproduce oppressive power dynamics is a vital part of politicizing neuronormativity. To work within a neurodiversity paradigm approach, then, this understanding and awareness must be built into everything from study design in scientific research to policies regarding the ways schools and workplaces are organized. As we will further clarify throughout this book, this is necessary for improving our theory, research, and practice in ways that are neurodivergence-inclusive.

Taking the two core principles of affirming complexity and politicizing neuronormativity helps us remain aware of how different forms of oppression often intersect. The neurodiversity paradigm will fail if it aims at neurodivergent liberation only, rather than collective liberation more generally. This means that to make the neurodiversity paradigm effective, its proponents also need to commit to other liberatory struggles.

Chapter 2
Neurodiversity as democratic theory and research

In the previous chapter we began to introduce what we might call 'neurodiversity theory'. This refers to the body of theory associated with the neurodiversity movement. In this chapter we will cover core components of the theory in more detail, with a particular focus on models of disability, the very idea of the 'normal' mind or brain, and the nature of neurominorities and controversies around diagnosis. This by no means covers all of neurodiversity, but these are core themes that are helpful for beginning with.

While we cover several different themes, something we want to emphasize throughout is that in the neurodiversity movement we see a shift towards a democratic approach to theory and research. By this we mean a shift away from viewing knowledge, and the practices we base on this, being constructed by a relatively small number of (usually neurotypical) experts, and towards a broader understanding of expertise as dispersed across our neurologically diverse populations. We take this shift towards greater democracy as following from the core neurodiversity paradigm principles of affirming complexity and politicizing neuronormativity, since democracy is always an attempt to navigate the complexities of political issues. It is notable here that a slogan of the Disability Rights movement, as well as of struggles for Black liberation, has long been *nothing about us without us*. With this in mind, the notion of neurodiversity theory as a shift towards a more democratic approach, which emphasizes the need to centre neurodivergent voices, is a thread that we will use throughout this chapter to help clarify how the various themes we cover interrelate. Towards the end of the chapter, we will shift from theory to research, to show how a more democratic approach might help change empirical knowledge production in line with the principles of the neurodiversity paradigm.

Models of disability

Disability is the general term used for whenever someone has a body or mind that is considered impaired, and which is associated with struggling to fulfil the usual expectations of society. This includes expectations in school, the workplace, in day-to-day activities, and so on. Disabilities may in some cases also be associated with disease or illness, while in other cases someone can be disabled but healthy. They can also be permanent, temporary, or sporadic states. Legal definitions also differ in different contexts, and what is officially recognized as a disability thus slightly changes in different times and places.

Beyond definitions, our understandings of and responses to disability can change dramatically depending on which model of disability we adopt. Disability models are a bit like different lenses that we can use to understand disability, each of which comes with different assumptions and commitments. This is relevant for neurodiversity theory since the neurodiversity paradigm challenges the dominant way of viewing neurological disabilities and suggests different ways of viewing them. Historically, moral or religious models of disability have often dominated. These saw disability as caused by supernatural forces: a disability might be viewed as a punishment from a god, or an opportunity for moral growth. But in the modern era we have shifted towards a more medical and scientific approach. This rejects the idea of disability as a moral issue and instead views it naturalistically, as a problem of the body or mind to be prevented or corrected through scientifically based medical intervention. We will explain this before going on to alternative models that we associate more with the neurodiversity movement.

The basic idea of the *medical model* is that bodily or mental impairment or dysfunction is what causes illness or disability—you may recognize this as this model goes hand-in-hand with the normalcy paradigm we have already described, but has more direct implications for practice. Namely, that to respond to disability or illness appropriately means trying to prevent, treat, or cure underlying impairments or dysfunctions. Since the early 19th century at least, medical science and practice have been geared towards this, primarily through the use of genetic, physiological, or psychological intervention. As a result, autism or ADHD, bipolar disorder or schizophrenia have traditionally been seen as individual medical problems to be corrected by therapy or biomedical intervention.

The medical model has been a significant improvement on the moral model in a range of ways. First, it avoids the stigma of viewing disability or illness as moral *failure*, and it also avoids pressuring disabled people (or their carers) to see their disability or illness as a chance for moral *growth*—a chance to be virtuous or inspirational while bearing great suffering. More importantly still, the medical model has often been hugely successful at preventing, treating, or curing a variety of illnesses or disabilities. Vaccines, antibiotics, and surgery, not to mention public health, sanitation, and so on, have radically reduced human suffering and increased the average lifespan considerably. All of this is in part the product of adopting and developing a medical model approach over the previous few centuries.

Despite the many benefits the medical model is associated with, it also has significant limitations and has brought its own harms. One issue is that the medical model tends to frame disability as an inherent tragedy, especially in cases where there is no effective treatment or cure. This can bring a kind of stigma of its own, leading disabled people to be viewed as inferior or as objects of pity. As a part of this, disabled people who achieve impressive things—including a degree of what is considered 'normal', such as having a job—are viewed as inspirational, something which disability advocates routinely reject. Relatedly, only focusing on deficits can also often lead to overlooking positives associated with many forms of neurodivergence. In the worst-case scenario, which is rather common, any difference between a neurodivergent and neurotypical person is immediately classified as a neurodivergent deficit. Finally, disabled people have argued that many of their key problems do not stem primarily from their impairments, but rather from societal exclusion, discrimination, and barriers. From their perspective, the medical model overlooks this, and thereby contributes to depoliticizing disablement.

Because of the failures of the medical model, in the 1970s radical disability activists proposed what came to be called the social model of disability. This model is only about disability rather than illness, and it distinguishes between impairment (of the body or mind) and disablement. Based on this, instead of assuming that disability always stems directly from an impairment, it suggests a different story, whereby disablement is caused primarily by societal barriers. For instance, a wheelchair user with mobility impairments will be excluded from participation in society when access is via steps but not ramps, when dropped pavements are blocked by inconsiderate parking, when public toilets are not built to accommodate them, or when airlines lose or damage their wheelchair. This shifts the emphasis away from viewing disablement simply as an apolitical, individual problem to be fixed by medical intervention. Instead, disabled people are recast as an oppressed group, in need of rights, justice, and liberation no less than some are in need of access to medical treatment.

The understanding that disabled people are both oppressed and marginalized has permitted attention to be paid to the role of minority stress in the lives of disabled—and more specifically, neurodivergent—people. Minority stress describes the forms of stress particularly experienced as a result of being part of a minority group, in a given society. Minority stress arises in part from phenomena like discrimination and prejudice-driven aggression, but is also present in the absence of these, as a direct result of being 'other than' the majority. Recognizing the experience and effects of minority stress is a crucial part of working towards neurodivergent liberation and directly flows from the social model of disability which recasts disabled people as a societal minority.

The original social model of disability (and its variants, since many theorists have since suggested various tweaks or additions to this basic conceptualization) has been a powerful tool for disabled people to fight for rights and justice in recent decades. This was also one of the key theoretical tools that neurodiversity proponents adopted from the 1990s onward. For instance, this allowed autistic people to begin seeing their sensory processing problems as stemming in large part from the neurotypical-biased design of schools, workplaces, and so on. Similarly, it allowed the insight that dyslexic people's struggles in the classroom could be viewed as stemming in significant part from the neuronormative focus on writing and texts rather than speech and audio, or problems in timing on exams, and so on. Based on this, neurodiversity proponents have been able to successfully challenge the neuronormative ways much of the world is structured.

The social model has also allowed a shift away from viewing disability as an individual tragedy. Some disabled people have even cultivated conceptions of disability pride, analogous to gay pride. Most relevantly, when it comes to neurodiversity, this includes notions of Autistic pride, Mad pride, and Weird pride. These indicate celebrations of Mad and Autistic culture, community, and solidarity. This has been extremely empowering for many neurodivergent people and has helped challenge overly negative perceptions of neurodivergence left over from the medical model.

It should be noted here that not all disabled people fully embrace the social model. Some suggest that it leads to overlooking the harmful effects of impairments, and some feel the medical model better fits with aspects of their experience. Because of this, some disability theorists have proposed *relational models* (or interactional models) that seek to provide a middle ground. Instead of committing to the idea that disability stems either from the impairment (within the person) or from society (outside the person), relational models view it as stemming from a complex interaction between individual bodyminds and the world. Moreover, the extent to which any given individual's disability stems from one or the other will be different in different cases. These models thus seek to provide more space for a wider range of disabilities, drawing on the most beneficial aspects of both medicalized and social approaches. Other theorists have simply supplemented the social model with the concept of 'impairment effects', which can be acknowledged even while viewing disability as a more general political problem.

The neurodiversity movement has been influenced by both social and relational models, and either is compatible with the neurodiversity approach. While they do not deny the utility of a medical approach in many instances, by shifting the focus onto how society excludes and disables neurodivergent people, they have combated overly negative and pathologizing approaches to neurodivergent disablement and distress. Adopting and updating the insights of social and relational models of disability is thus a key part of neurodiversity theory.

Standpoint epistemology

A related shift that is at least implicit in much neurodiversity advocacy is a shift in epistemology. Epistemology refers to theories of knowledge, which are particularly relevant when it comes to understanding what might constitute expertise about neurodivergence. The medical model draws on a theory of knowledge that positions medical researchers, clinicians, and physicians as the experts. Their specialist training and access to scientific knowledge is considered to give them unique capacity when it comes not just to understanding disability, but also how to respond to it. These assumptions are reinforced by anxieties in biomedical sciences about 'bias' as a consequence of subjectivity. Much of biomedical research methodology is designed to recognize and eliminate sources of bias, most notably in systematic reviews and clinical trials. A number of international registration and reporting systems are now in place to enforce these anti-bias measures. In this context, the idea that an individual, or a group of people with some degree of shared lived experience, might have not just privileged insight but valuable expertise is hard for some to recognize.

This is challenged, although not wholly rejected, by neurodiversity proponents. As we have just discussed, by shifting to a social model of disability, neurodiversity proponents also make the shift to viewing disabled people as forming an oppressed class, with more specific disabilities forming more specific classes. Looked at this way, it becomes possible to emphasize how disabled people may have special insight into their own positioning, and how this impacts their lives, that outsiders do not have. Thus, a doctor may have specific knowledge about, say, the scientific literature on a given disability, but a disabled person will have their own life experiences, and often also community knowledge, making them an expert too. This community knowledge becomes both more scientifically valuable and politically influential when it forms a collective cultural understanding. Sharing and combining experiences to extrapolate cultural norms for neurodivergent people, or for a specific group within that, helps to generate authoritative statements about 'the ADHD experience' that can shape practice while being resilient to the effects of individual agendas or bias.

When we relate this back to affirming complexity and politicizing neuronormativity, this helps us see why we say that neurodiversity proponents can be seen as pushing for a more democratic approach. The shift to what some social theorists refer to as *standpoint epistemology* emphasizes that all knowledge comes from one specific standpoint or another, and moreover that members of oppressed classes often have insights into their oppression that will be missed from outside. As applied to neurodivergence, this does not deny that non-disabled doctors and researchers can contribute relevant expert knowledge, but it also emphasizes that in other ways they will often be ignorant. By the same token, disabled people also have their own expertise, but may be ignorant about various other things, such as the potential side effects of a given medication. Even for this superficially clear example, though, the doctor's authority is not absolute. We know that medications can work differently for some neurodivergent people, and this might not be apparent from clinical trial data where neurodivergence is not taken into account. Thus, neurodivergent people may have situated knowledge from their community that doctors might lack. This will be different in every case, not least because disabled people and doctors are not mutually exclusive categories. Moreover, many disabled people may also be multiply marginalized, and will thus have access to experiences and knowledge that may be missed by disabled people who are not multiply marginalized. Given all of this, the neurodiversity paradigm shifts to a more democratic approach to knowledge production. That is, it emphasizes that our understandings must be developed collectively, and this goes for anything from theory to empirical research.

The concept of health and the normal mind

An important issue raised by the neurodiversity movement and its challenge to the normalcy paradigm regards how we understand what it means to be healthy or ill. It should be emphasized that the concept of health, as well as related concepts such as disease, illness, pathology, and so on, are continually and constantly contested. There has never been a single, universally accepted definition of any of these, and understandings change in different cultures, times, and places. Still, it is notable that all cultures globally have at least some conception of mental and physical health. Ancient medical texts from Egypt, India, Greece, and China, for instance, all document conceptions of health that are applied to both body and mind.

While concepts of health have changed over time, what is most important for neurodiversity theory is that health became more associated with normality in the 19th century in Europe. This was partly following the industrial revolution, which required bodies and minds to be standardized in relation to machines and products. It was also partly because modern statistical analysis was being developed, which allowed this standardization to be formalized through the use of data collection and analysis of mathematical averages and normal distributions.

While this has been helpful for the development of medical science in a number of ways, it has also arguably become harmful. The key issue with associating health with normality is that anyone who is atypical and struggling in any way is also seen as being disordered or having a pathology to be treated or cured. Sometimes this is helpful. In the case of epilepsy, for instance, most people with the condition want to be treated, and many would like to be cured if that ever becomes possible. But in other cases, it is harmful. Until the 1980s it was wrongly thought that homosexuality was a mental disorder. Because lots of queer people struggle with mental health problems and since queerness is atypical, psychiatrists came to believe that queerness itself was a disorder that should be treated medically. But this only harmed queer people, and now we recognize that high levels of mental health problems in queer populations are related to the stigma and discrimination queer people face.

This means that a big part of combating the normalcy paradigm regards the need to cleave the conceptual link between health and normality. At the moment, it is not totally clear what, if any, single conception of health the neurodiversity paradigm is committed to. After all, neurodiversity proponents do tend to retain some conception of mental or neurological illness (e.g. for epilepsy or dementia), even while contesting others. Reconceptualizing what it means to be healthy is a key task for neurodiversity theory, and more work will need to be done on this over the coming decades. At the same time, it should be noted that since nobody has proposed a perfect definition of health, the fact that neurodiversity proponents don't have one is not a reason to dismiss the neurodiversity paradigm. It only means that neurodiversity proponents need to grapple with a problem that is equally a problem for everyone else.

For now, one way of thinking about the neurodiversity paradigm approach to theorizing health—and the boundaries between health and pathology—again might consist in democratizing how we approach this. At the moment, for instance, a great many autistic people contest that autism is non-pathological. By contrast, there is nothing like this collective position (yet) in relation to obsessive-compulsive disorder, indicating that most people with OCD see it as a pathological condition. In the neurodiversity movement the emphasis has most often been on allowing atypical people and groups to decide for themselves whether they consider their divergences pathological or not. This can be seen as the beginning of a more democratic approach to determining which forms of divergence are healthy or pathological, rather than our standards being enforced through an equivalence between health and normal functioning.

Neurodiversity and diagnostic categories

Since the standard way to recognize disability is currently clinical diagnosis, it is vital to consider diagnosis in more detail. Moreover, understanding how the neurodiversity paradigm relates to diagnostic systems of classification is essential to the goals both of affirming complexity and politicizing neuronormativity. Our overarching position is that neurodiversity is fully aligned with a process of identification of disability, or divergence, but that this process should be maximally democratized and should serve the needs of the people who attract diagnosis, not just those who assess them. In the longer term, we suggest, a neurodiversity paradigm approach should work towards building a world where independent, formal clinical diagnosis is not always necessary for recognition of disability.

The first thing to establish is that psychiatric diagnostic classification systems, namely the Diagnostic and Statistical Manual of Mental Disorders (currently DSM-5) and the International Classification of Diseases (currently ICD-11), are created by humans to serve human purposes. The explicit rationale for psychiatric diagnoses is that this is necessary for people to access appropriate support or treatment, not to mention for other things such as health insurance and employment rights. They often do function in this way, for instance, accessing ADHD medications or psychotherapy. For many, diagnoses are also helpful for self-understanding and are preferable to more stigmatizing labels they might otherwise receive ('lazy', 'naughty', etc.). Many also find diagnoses useful for finding communities of other neurodivergent people who share their experiences.

At the same time, however, such classifications can also serve purposes of social control. As we have already highlighted, being gay or lesbian used to be pathologized as a mental disorder (and in some countries still is); women resisting patriarchy have been labelled as hysterical or as having disordered personalities; Black civil rights protesters were pathologized as having a 'protest psychosis'. Still today, diagnosis can be used to deny support as much as to provide it, and moreover some diagnoses increase stigma. In such cases, the label is not serving the needs of the patient. As across all medicine, then, diagnosis can range from being life-saving to lethal depending on how it is used, and which societal functions it serves.

A deeper issue regards the relationship between the map and the territory, and to what extent diagnoses reflect discoveries or inventions. Many clinicians and researchers would like to believe that the diagnostic categories we have derived from observing human behaviour possess a degree of natural authority, or ground truth: that we are not *inventing*, but instead *discovering* classifications which are pre-existing. In some cases of neurodivergence, there seems a stronger case for this. The classification of Down syndrome, for instance, based on a single and specific genetic feature, seems closer to a discovery than other, much vaguer classifications with more shifting boundaries.

However, viewing diagnoses as fixed or static—and using overly simple binaries between discovery and invention—goes against the neurodiversity paradigm commitments to affirming complexity and politicizing neuronormativity. For the most part, while the human race may be infinitely diverse, often this diversity does not fall into substantively different classes with clear space in between. Increasingly, transdiagnostic research is providing robust scientific support for this position. For example, in one analysis, authors identified 628 symptoms that make up all adult psychopathology described in the DSM-5. Of these, over one-third of the listed symptoms appear in more than one diagnostic classification. The most common number of repeats is for a symptom to appear in three separate diagnoses, but the range spans from 2 to 22 repeat appearances. In other words, in psychiatry, overlap is the norm rather than the exception when it comes to diagnostic classification. Similarly, in research examining neurodevelopmental diversity in children, a number of studies have found it is possible to cluster children, by shared genetics, shared neurological features, shared cognitive profiles, or shared diagnoses. But importantly none of these clustering systems maps across levels—children with the same diagnosis do not consistently share a cognitive, neurological, or genetic signature. Indeed, even Down syndrome has broad variation in terms of the community's cognitive profiles, and how it is framed and represented is often a social as much as a natural matter.

If diagnoses often do not represent the formalized endpoint of a process of discovery of underlying truths, then what do they represent? One possibility is that, even when we put aside misuse of diagnoses to enforce patriarchal, heteronormative, or white supremacist ends, diagnostic classifications themselves often serve the purpose of enforcing neuronormativity and carve the world up into groups in order to control us. They may do this both by separating people into categories and by attempting to impose a degree of uniformity (or presumed uniformity) within a category. In this sense, current diagnosis systems, at least insofar as they present their classifications as representing discrete, natural dysfunctions, seem out of step with the neurodiversity paradigm.

As well as this fundamental mismatch, there are also practical ways in which the current diagnostic hegemony stands in the way of the long-term goals of the neurodiversity movement. In research, diagnostic classifications dominate when it comes to participant recruitment and to measurement of relevant characteristics or phenomena. Case-control methods in which highly selective criteria are applied, and measures chosen based on pre-existing understandings of what is interesting about a given population (in ADHD, executive functions; in autism, social cognition; in dyslexia, verbal IQ), can limit our capacity to capture rich insights into neurodivergent experiences and outcomes. These problems are exacerbated by the desire to find significant differences between groups, which are more achievable when those groups are narrowly defined—for example by excluding people who are multiply neurodivergent. These approaches create artificial clear space between diagnoses, exaggerating differences and obscuring shared features.

Another issue worth noting is that, in education and services, the absolute authority of clinical diagnosis frequently acts as a gatekeeper to support—as when children require a diagnosis before support in the classroom or during assessments will be considered. This has practical detriment, as people wait to be seen by clinical services before action is taken to alleviate difficulties. The problems can become severe when diagnostic services are overwhelmed, as at the time of writing in the UK, in the wake of the Covid-19 pandemic. Diagnostic gatekeeping drives inequality as well, in the light of known differentials in access to diagnosis based on social class, ethnicity, and gender.

This problem is not just practical, but also existential, as waiting for clinical diagnosis can limit people's potential for self-actualization, via recognition of this element of their identity. By endorsing a diagnostic system governed by clinical professionals and their manuals, we devalue the knowledge of the person who perceives their own neurodivergence, instead focusing on external validation. What does it mean that neurodivergent people do not necessarily feel able to self-identify, that their insight into their own experience of the world is secondary to the judgement of an outsider? The reification of the authority of clinicians is so influential that even within neurodivergent communities the concept of self-identification (as autistic, dyspraxic, having ADHD) is frequently challenged, with people refusing to accept an individual into a community setting unless they have the authority of a clinical diagnosis.

A final problem with our diagnosis system is the way that the concept of diagnosis is colloquially understood. Diagnosis happens most commonly in relation to disease and is normally followed by an effort at a cure. While many patients will seek a diagnosis in the presence of symptoms—meaning the condition was pre-existing—nonetheless the point of diagnosis often marks a transition from being understood as healthy to unhealthy, and the beginning of a process to return to the former state. Of course, seeking to treat a neurodivergent medical condition is sometimes helpful, as in the case of motor neurone disease. But in other cases, identifying neurodivergent disability should really be an experience of uncovering a lifelong way of being, rather than being viewed as a matter of detecting a pathology to be treated.

Given all of this, do we call for the wholesale rejection of diagnosis as a system? We remain more ambivalent to diagnosis. One thing that neurodiversity proponents have done highly successfully is reclaim diagnoses, challenging how they are represented, understood, and studied. Many neurodivergent people identify as such, or simply as Mad, regardless of whether this has been certified by a doctor. Some neurodivergent people such as Merri Lisa Johnson have reclaimed diagnoses such as borderline personality. The reasoning here partly relies on the shift to standpoint epistemology and recognition of disabled people as forming marginalized groups in an oppressed class, as we have reviewed previously. Neurodivergent activists have also made their own classifications, such as 'AuDHD', which indicates an intersection between autism and ADHD. In line with politicizing neuronormativity, such classifications are then used as a basis for community, culture, and campaigning towards liberatory struggles. Thus while the neurodiversity paradigm seems at odds with much diagnostic practice in its current form, and certainly has room for alternatives to diagnosis, it is not clear that it requires abolition of diagnosis as such. Rather, it requires the abolition of diagnostic categories used in the service of domination and oppression.

With all this in mind, the overarching move we suggest, which comes with a neurodiversity approach, follows the more general theme of democratizing theory and research. In clinical diagnostic services, this transition requires recognition of standpoint epistemology: that all knowledge production is constrained by the standpoint of the individual. This epistemological shift should require a clinically trained practitioner to recognize the biases and limitations of their perspective and respectfully integrate them with the perspective of the person seeking a diagnosis. More generally, a shift to democratization of diagnosis should reject the hierarchy of doctor/patient and start to facilitate accurate and helpful self-identification.

Crucially, this democratization should extend to the classification system itself. Currently, the way medical diagnostic categories are made is through consensus conferences and voting among taskforces primarily made up of psychiatrists and other doctors. This means that there is some level of democracy, but if so, it is a very partial democracy, analogous to early Greek conceptions of democracy whereby only property-owning males of noble birth were able to vote. By contrast, a neurodiversity paradigm approach indicates the need to radically democratize classificatory processes, placing the perspectives of disabled people more centrally than those of clinicians or researchers. This would allow categories and labels that form the diagnostic structures to serve the needs of neurodivergent people, rather than the needs of the medical industrial complex.

At first glance, this might seem unachievable, but there are many examples of shifts already taking place which are moving towards a more democratized diagnostic framework. One partial shift occurred when the major diagnostic manuals removed the restriction that ADHD could not be diagnosed in the presence of an existing autism diagnosis. This had meant it was literally impossible for a clinician to diagnose ADHD and autism in the same person, meaning that diagnoses served the system's desire for clean categorical boundaries far more than the patient's need to be understood and to understand themselves. Another shift took place in the diagnostic criteria for autism, when the requirement for symptoms to be present in early development was softened to include recognition that they 'may not become fully manifest until social demands exceed limited capacities, or may be masked by learned strategies in later life' in DSM-5. Notably, this change was driven by the Autistic Self-Advocacy Network, who lobbied the American Psychiatric Association while they were updating diagnostic categories, forcing the classification to reflect the needs of autistic communities rather than centring clinician standpoints. This change in the language of diagnostic manuals is now being extended even further in diagnostic practice, as individual clinicians shift their understanding of their role away from identifying clinical 'impairment' and towards identifying characteristic patterns of behaviour and experience—thus expanding access to diagnosis and uplifting the authority of the patient. Finally, there is the mass shift towards self-identification already noted. While clinical diagnosis is often vital, for instance for accessing prescriptions or ruling out underlying neurological problems, the general shift towards self-identification is indicative of the beginnings of a mass democratizing process in how our classifications are made and used.

Applications in scientific research

Academic research provides the foundations for policy and practice within nations and globally, by generating conceptual models of understanding and providing a direct evidence base. Therefore, the goals of the neurodiversity movement—or the application of the neurodiversity paradigm—require a neurodiversity-affirmative research culture as well.

As it stands, research across disciplines is rife with examples of academic enquiry that directly contravene the neurodiversity paradigm, and instead serve to promote ableism and stigma and entrench or pursue neuronormativity. The long association of autism with a lack of empathy (now refuted) has been used in arguments about the extent to which empathy is a requirement of being human, implicitly and sometimes explicitly calling into question the humanity of autistic people. In psychological sciences, when we look across studies comparing neurodivergent with neurotypical participants we see that opposing group differences (e.g. in one study neurotypical brains have fewer

connections, in another the connections are more dense) are
routinely interpreted as indicating a deficit in the neurodivergent
group. In biomedical sciences, vast quantities of research funding
and researcher time are invested in a quest for biomarkers that
will reify diagnostic categories and could potentially be used as
part of a prenatal screening programme—something which is
already widespread for Down syndrome.

How instead might we deliver a research programme, across
disciplines, that could be considered neurodiversity affirmative?
The first and primary component of such research is the
involvement of neurodivergent people in leadership and
decision-making roles. This remains vanishingly rare—even
those fields where participatory methods are most established
mostly deliver consultations, where neurodivergent input is
constrained and channelled. A key way to improve this
situation is to cultivate greater neurodivergent representation
in academia, so that neurodivergent people are seeking
funding, delivering projects, publishing papers, and
shaping impact themselves.

Even if we achieve greater inclusion for neurodivergent people
in academia, this does not negate the need for participatory
methods—such as co-production, citizen science, and community
partnership—in research. Neurodivergent people who become
academics will always represent a subset of this complex and
heterogeneous community. Indeed, the process of becoming an
academic, studying for a PhD, and pursuing a career in the higher
education sector will shape neurodivergent academics in such a
way that they will inevitably be set apart from a range of key
neurodivergent experiences. Thus, neurodivergent academics are
not exempt from the requirement to engage with the community
and find ways to democratize their research process.

One example of a neurodiversity affirmative research programme,
manifest across multiple disciplines and research teams around

the globe, is research into the *double empathy problem.* First described by Damian Milton, the double empathy problem provides a neat encapsulation of the experience of communication breakdown that can occur between two people of different neurological persuasions. The idea was developed particularly to describe the social experiences of autistic people, and to challenge the interpretation that any communication or interactive challenges experienced between autistic and non-autistic people should be attributed to an impairment within the autistic person. Instead, the double empathy problem highlights that responsibility for the success of an interaction sits with both people involved, and that two interacting people may both need to make an effort to overcome a mismatch in communication style.

The double empathy problem has now given rise to a wealth of academic research, examining it from a theoretical, social science, experimental, and experiential perspective. Examples of this include seminal work demonstrating that non-autistic people make negative snap-judgements about autistic people, based on minimal information. Others have shown that the long-established difficulty that autistic people have (on average) judging the emotional facial expressions of others goes in both directions. Non-autistic people also struggle accurately to judge the emotional reactions of autistic people. Catherine Crompton captured the social experiences of autistic people in autistic and non-autistic company through interviews, systematically showing what many autistic people have long noted—that the company of other autistic people is comfortable and rewarding. In later experimental work she built on these findings, directly assessing how information was transferred between autistic, non-autistic, or mixed pairs of people. Her examinations of these interactions revealed that information transfer was more effective, and rapport was higher for matched pairs—both when rated by the participants themselves and by external observers.

Another example of research that affirms complexity, in a very literal sense, is the rise of transdiagnostic studies of development. This is a major departure from a long history of studies in which children are recruited to fit a set of narrow inclusion criteria. Not only selected for their diagnostic status—having ADHD, Tourette's syndrome, or dyslexia—but also required not to have any secondary diagnoses, intellectual disability, physical disabilities, and so on. By including a carefully filtered selection of children, in pursuit of the maximum possible difference between included groups, these studies can only serve to showcase homogeneity within a group and clear space between groups, thereby reinforcing neuronormativity. In contrast, studies like the CALM cohort in Cambridge, UK, and the POND database in Montreal, Canada, are open to a diverse range of children and teenagers. They are producing insights about how children develop, learn, and thrive which have the potential to showcase and gain insights into neurodiversity—though such work is not automatically or fully neurodiversity affirmative.

Applications in the arts and humanities

The influence of neurodiversity in academia is by no means limited to the sciences. A significant part of neurodiversity theory can be seen as part of the discipline of philosophy, and thus we might speak of there being a sub-field of philosophy of neurodiversity. This also has a lot of overlap with the component of disability studies often called disability theory. Much of what we have already covered regarding the basics of neurodiversity theory could be described as part of disability theory or philosophy of disability. This includes, most notably, analysis of the fundamental concepts and theoretical positions associated with the movement, which are more primarily conceptual than scientific matters.

But neurodiversity theory equally relates to a range of other disciplines in the arts and humanities. For a start, we could speak of critical neurodiversity theory, which is less about the metaphysical basis of the paradigm and is more about understanding neurodiversity in relation to society as a whole. The point of this is to theorize neurodivergent oppression in relation to broader systems of oppression and historical conditions, in order to think more clearly about what neurodivergent liberation might require.

Neurodiversity theory also has important implications for a range of other disciplines in the arts and humanities. Consider history. Most of our current historical work on things like Tourette's syndrome or ADHD has been developed through a normalcy paradigm lens. Beginning with the assumptions of the normalcy paradigm will inevitably lead to certain interpretations of history which may be different from those developed through a neurodiversity paradigm lens. This may include anything from interpretations of Shakespeare to the history of capitalism. As such it is important to retell our histories through the neurodiversity paradigm, emphasizing how neuronormativity and the scientific research and clinical practice relating to this has always been political.

Similarly, neurodiversity theory may also inform disciplines that are engaged in cultural critique, such as literary studies, art history, theatre studies, and film and television studies. Until recently, engagement with neurodiversity in these fields tended to focus on questions of authenticity and the politics of representation: how do we decide what 'good' depictions of neurodivergence look like? Who gets to make this judgement? Should neurotypical persons be able to portray neurodivergent characters in film/theatre/television? Can neurotypical authors depict neurodivergence in literature in a non-pathologizing way? It is important that we ask these questions of contemporary media if we are to enact the tenets of the neurodiversity paradigm and its emphasis on self-definition and creating equitable relationships and understandings across neurotypes.

However, when working with texts or other cultural products that were produced prior to our current understandings of neurodiversity (or of specific diagnoses), scholars caution against the tempting practice of fictional and/or historical diagnosis. The reason for this is that, even when the intention might be to find kinship with fictional characters, the practice of identifying certain characters as autistic, for example, replicates the practices of a culture that seeks to pathologize difference. Relatedly, when we are dealing with fictional constructs, we cannot assume that the established neurological normative of a given text reflects the understanding of its publication contexts. There must always be space to reflect upon the use of neurodivergence as a metaphorical device or as a carrier of cultural critique, rather than a straightforward representation of lived experience. Louise Creechan observes that 'neurodivergence' is an implicitly relational term that responds to the normative standard as established within a text which may or may not align with 'real-world' categorizations. By this schema, a neurodiversity framework might be applied to texts from any historical period or to the speculative or imaginative worlds of science fiction or fantasy. This form of analysis focuses, not on accuracy, but on the dynamics and tensions created by neurological variation within literary texts. Scholars working at the intersection of critical autism studies and literature have considered the interpretive potential of autistic readership and autistic poetics in literary texts, but these analyses have maintained the pathologizing parameters of autism diagnosis.

As the neurodiversity paradigm advocates for valuing and engaging with the natural diversity of minds, it is perhaps unsurprising that neurodiversity scholarship in the arts and humanities is often deeply invested in questions of form. Neurodivergent artists and activists have sought to redefine the traditions of live performance to accommodate variations in bodyminds, as explored by the contributors to *Awkwoods* and in Jess Thom's (aka Touretteshero) tourettic, relaxed performances of Samuel Beckett's *Not I*. Similarly, neurodivergent scholars and artists have advocated for forms of scholarship that capitalize upon the inclusive potentialities of mixed media, such as zines and collage. Through embracing and valuing a variety of mediums, atypical bodyminds can forge their access to scholarship in their own terms.

Neurodiversity theory thus has great relevance for a range of humanities fields, and an important part of the paradigm shift will require developing new knowledges within these fields to help reposition neurodivergent people in the past and today. This also relates to the wider attempt at a cultural paradigm, which relates to but goes far beyond academic research, and can be seen in myriad forms of neurodivergent art and literature that are being produced by neurodivergent artists.

A general orientation of this effort, and a key way to live up to the principles of affirming complexity and politicizing neuronormativity, is a mass push towards democratizing research, all the way from how we construct our categories to the way we design studies, the questions we ask, and so forth. By democratizing we mean moving away from primarily centring the efforts of a few experts, and instead developing knowledge through and with neurodiverse populations in ways that situate the needs of neurodivergent people over the needs of research. The ultimate point of this is to redirect our theory and research towards changing the world in ways that will be good for neurodivergent people everywhere.

Chapter 3
Applications of the neurodiversity paradigm

In this chapter we will move on from theory to practice, discussing applications of the neurodiversity approach in education, the workplace, the criminal justice system, and health and social care. To be clear, this is by no means meant to be exhaustive, but these are some of the key areas where developing a neurodiversity paradigm approach has the most potential for impact. These themes also allow us to take a lifespan approach, since our lives typically begin by entering the education system, we then typically move on to or are shut out of the workplace—and, in some cases, may encounter the criminal justice system—and finally, we all need health and social care, and many of us end up in nursing homes. As such, though there is no standard trajectory for any single life, these themes allow us to uncover some issues that neurodivergent people might directly or indirectly encounter.

Before beginning this section, it is important to recognize that the systems and tools used to build current practices, evaluate them, and improve them are themselves potentially neuronormative. As we have mentioned, academic research which supports national and local policy change and also shapes the decisions of individuals (e.g. a headteacher deciding how to spend their pupil support budget in a given year; a clinical service lead making induction materials for new staff) is not an accessible space for many neurodivergent people. Growing numbers of neurodivergent academics describe the challenges and costs of their chosen career, while others only survive by keeping their neurodivergence carefully hidden. At a deeper level, the very tools with which knowledge is constructed are grounded in neuronormative expectations about the nature of evidence and indicators of rigour—as in the title of Audre Lorde's seminal work *The Master's Tools Will Never Dismantle the Master's House.* In that context, we call for a degree of epistemic disobedience—willingness to challenge the orthodoxy at all levels—when it comes to developing new understandings to support radical shifts in practice across society.

Being neurodivergent in school

The modern, inclusive school system, of the kind laid down in UNESCO and UNICEF guidelines, is where many neurodivergent people first encounter regular discrimination and exclusion. This means that we must change education if we want to shift to a broader neurodiversity paradigm. In this section we will cover the basics of the current system to show some more general issues as well as what it might mean to shift to a neurodiversity-affirmative approach.

An inclusive education system means that efforts are made to provide a single school setting which caters to a diverse range of young people. However, inclusion is rarely complete. First, those pupils with the most significant learning disabilities, making traditional learning methods and targets inappropriate for them, are usually educated separately in 'special schools'—though the terminology varies. Second, many mainstream schools which accommodate neurotypical and neurodivergent children will also have an attached 'learning support base' or similar. This is intended to give neurodivergent young people the chance to move flexibly between mainstream classrooms and a more tailored learning environment, catering to so-called 'spikey profiles' of ability and variations in capacity depending on other factors. Such

bases may also be used by children with English as an additional
language, or those who have experienced significant trauma.
Third, exclusion of neurodivergent pupils from mainstream school
is common. Young people may be formally excluded, but even
more common are hidden exclusions, which we will describe in
more detail below. Finally, anxiety-related school non-attendance
and home-schooling is prevalent in families of a neurodivergent
child, meaning many have opted out of the state school system,
finding it unfit for their needs.

Debates about the application of the neurodiversity paradigm in
schools must first recognize two things. First, that the goal of
inclusive education—well established as a principle worldwide—is
inclusion. Specifically, by this we mean that the success of an
inclusive education system rests on how well it has managed to
include diverse learners. This is distinct from attainment goals,
which are often the focus in the classroom, against which some
learners will always fail. Attainment goals matter for capitalist
societies, where a key purpose of education is preparing young
people to enter the job market. Modern education systems
typically include mandatory schooling up to a certain point and
then optional further education beyond that. Since the 19th
century, much learning and assessment in modern school systems
has become increasingly standardized. This is supposed to be fair,
allowing everyone to be trained and tested in the same way as
everyone else. This is why we tend to have standard tests, a
standardized curriculum, and so on, used across nations of many
millions of people. However, these rigid systems serve a set of
capitalist workforce demands (at least for the subset of pupils
who meet expectations), but not the goal of inclusion.

The second acknowledgement is that traditionally a key purpose
of a country's education system is to socialize children to the
norms and expectations of their cultural context and especially of
the workplace. Children learn about rules, hierarchy, and peer
relationships as much as they learn spelling, fractions, and history.

This is important because it reminds us that an inclusive education system does not just consider access to formal learning, but also access and affirmation in a system of socialization.

Schools currently fail neurodivergent children across the board. A key issue is that standardized schooling excludes the ways many people function or process information. This means people with statistically rare skills or talents go unrecognized or may fail on tests designed for an imaginary typical student. This is often particularly hard for multiply marginalized neurodivergent people. For instance, a migrant student learning in a second language may diverge both neurologically and culturally from the imagined typical student, making it harder for them to gain access to both education and socialization processes throughout school. Another key issue is that learning and socialization may be especially hard given that schools are often chaotic, loud, and busy places. While this is challenging for nearly everyone, it can be highly detrimental to the processing styles of many neurodivergent people. Finally, schools may also often have rules and norms that are particularly harmful for neurodivergent people. For instance, having to sit still for long periods may be detrimental to the learning of students who fit with the ADHD diagnosis, or expectations in physical education classes may exclude some students with impaired bodily coordination, as is associated with a dyspraxia (or developmental coordination disorder) diagnosis.

All this means school is often a deeply traumatizing place for many neurodivergent people, especially those who are from working-class and minority ethnic backgrounds. Currently, neurodivergent children and young people are more likely to be excluded from school and have higher rates of non-attendance. They are also subject to unknown rates of 'hidden exclusions', such as parents being asked to collect their child before the end of the school day, pupils being excluded on external inspection dates, and pupils spending much of the day in isolation. When they do attend, they have lower participation in class and are more likely to be bullied and victimized. Some families may resort to seeking a placement for their child in a special school. For some neurodivergent people, where the mainstream learning environment is entirely inaccessible, special school placements are helpful and appropriate, but for many it is inadequate. Disabled learners should not have to seek out a placement which presumes less ability, simply in order to be accepted socially and accommodated behaviourally. In practice, desperate families seeking special education placements results in a form of segregation, where people with the same learning potential are divided up into a two-tier education system that perpetuates oppression more than reducing it.

These educational inequalities ripple out, contributing to poorer reported quality of life for neurodivergent youth and their families and driving high rates of teacher burnout and dropout from the profession. The effects are long term as well, with many neurodivergent young people following the school-to-prison pipeline and struggling to access higher or further education and employment. As so often in this text, comprehensive figures are just not known, with evidence coming from a patchwork of studies normally limited to examining one diagnostic group or another.

Neurodiversity-affirmative education

A different approach to education emphasizes inclusion. This indicates a commitment to changing how classrooms and education more broadly are organized so that they work for everyone, not just those who sit closer to the imagined standard student. Beyond being inclusive, education can also be emancipatory. In his influential book *Pedagogy of the Oppressed*, the Brazilian educator Paulo Freire emphasized that while socialization is often helpful, preparing students to conform to an unjust society just reproduces injustice. Instead, Freire suggested what he called a 'dialogical' approach where students and teachers generate shared understandings and knowledge together. This could include knowledge about how students themselves have been oppressed. This kind of education would not just prepare students to adjust to society as it is, but also to actively participate in challenging the more oppressive tendencies around them.

Neurodiversity-affirmative education systems should be a way to correct these distressing patterns by instead turning to inclusive and emancipatory approaches. Importantly, neurodiversity-affirmative education would help to realize the goals of inclusion by making adjustments not only to formal learning and attainment aspects of education, but also to the socialization agenda in schools. Neurodiversity-informed education should affirm complexity, by expecting and catering to heterogeneity in the student body (and staff) as a matter of course. A shift to talking of needs that are met or unmet could be a useful signal here—moving away from the concept that neurodivergent pupils' needs are 'special' or 'additional'. Goals should be set based on individual flourishing rather than being centred on normative behaviour. Schools should also politicize neuronormativity, by recognizing the social forces that dictate neurodivergent experiences, including stereotypes, stigma, discrimination, and prejudice, and work to actively fight these. In doing so, they can draw on the strength that comes from diversity by involving diverse teams in developing and delivering policy and practice.

Full realization of these principles could drive a pivot towards education as a mechanism of liberation, by educating marginalized people to develop the potential to change society themselves. This is deep inclusion, centring the needs of the excluded and prioritizing the battle against inequality. It requires fundamental and radical change. However, sticking within existing curriculum frameworks, we can still implement neurodiversity-affirmative practices.

Implementation of these principles might include a programme of actively teaching children the insight and self-advocacy skills needed to judge their own behavioural and learning needs and request support as needed. Resources such as a classroom visual timetable, or the option to wear noise-cancelling headphones, should be available to all and not doled out selectively to those with a doctor-provided permission slip (in the form of a diagnosis). Relaxing rules is also vital. For instance, students should not be forced to sit still for long periods and should be able to freely use toilet facilities whenever they need to. Teachers should seize every opportunity to celebrate diversity: for example, noting and cherishing the range of approaches taken to writing and illustrating a poem about autumn, rather than selecting the 'best' poems. Applying the principles of the neurodiversity paradigm in our schools (and lifelong learning institutions) should help us realize the goals of inclusion by making neurodivergent learners feel accepted and welcome in class. This goal is a prerequisite for both well-being and educational attainment to follow.

Finally, helping all students build a general awareness of neuronormative oppression is also vital for emancipatory education. As we have indicated, all too often, key problems neurodivergent people face throughout their lives begin in education before being transported to the workplace and other aspects of adult life. This means that education is also a key place where neurotypical people begin to learn to see themselves as superior to neurodivergent people, and neurodivergent children begin to internalize feelings of inferiority. Collectively building an awareness and understanding of such issues in the classroom, through a dialogical approach building knowledge between teacher and students, is most likely a vital step towards overcoming this. After all, the world of tomorrow will be made by the students of today, and this includes both neurotypical and neurodivergent students.

Applications in the workplace

It is always challenging to estimate what proportion of the world is neurodivergent, but we can be clear that for any given neurodivergent group, unemployment rates are higher than in the general population. Sample statistics include full- or part-time employment rates of just 34 per cent for adults with ADHD and 15 per cent for people with a learning disability. Meanwhile, reporting on the National Longitudinal Transition Study 2 in the USA, autistic employment is described as follows: 'While the rate increased steadily for individuals on the spectrum from 15 to 63%, it was always lower than the average rate for all disability groups, which increased from 54 to 91%.'

Most of us leave full-time education at some point in our youth, and the general expectation is that decades of paid employment will follow. While, as we describe below, the assumption that paid employment is the only or best way to spend your adult life needs to be challenged, neurodivergent people should certainly have the same right and opportunity to succeed in work as anyone else. Paid employment brings a number of benefits—social connection, daily routine, a chance to use your skills and be rewarded for that. Some would argue, following Marx, that fulfilling one's creative potential is part of what it means, fundamentally, to be human—just as a beaver builds dams, we work to create new things, use them, and share them. More practically, perhaps the biggest reason to ensure equal access to work is that being paid wages is a huge part of having self-determination and autonomy.

However, modern workplaces rarely acknowledge, let alone accommodate, neurodivergence—resulting in the low rates of employment already mentioned. Recruitment processes often exclude neurodivergent people in all kinds of ways; for example, some personality tests used in recruitment are remarkably similar to those used for diagnoses such as bipolar disorder, and while it would be illegal to directly discriminate on these grounds, the tests used in recruitment can act as a proxy for discriminating against people with various diagnoses. For those neurodivergent people who do find work, a large majority of workplaces have become enforcers of neuronormativity, by the scientific management of workers and their efficiency. In factories, call centres, and offices, in Starbucks, McDonald's, and Aldi, workers must do more with less. Even in the UK's largest employer, the National Health Service, many elements of patient care are allotted by time quota rather than being permitted whatever resource is needed for a careful clinical decision. Productivity is key, and this is anathema to a neurodivergence-informed system that allows for cognitive diversity. It is no wonder then that anyone for whom reading takes a little more time, or whose working memory relies on a chance to recheck instructions, will find modern workplaces inhospitable at best.

There are ways to apply the principles of the neurodiversity paradigm in the workplace, however. The concept of reasonable adjustments goes a long way towards affirming complexity, by placing a legal responsibility on employers to provide for the unique needs of their individual employees. If correctly implemented, this system should allow an employee to ask for support or resources to enable them to do their job. For someone with chronic back pain, this could be a specialized chair or standing desk, and for a neurodivergent person it might be speech-to-text software or a solo office.

Unfortunately, in reality, there is a wealth of reporting from neurodivergent and otherwise disabled people that the reasonable adjustments system is rarely applied as intended in law—or rather, fails to achieve the desired goal of inclusion. One factor that might particularly apply to neurodivergent people is a lack of clarity on what adjustments might be available and helpful for them. This is something that is frequently reported anecdotally and is not surprising given the relative invisibility of neurodivergent people in workplaces until very recently. Many neurodivergent people are not 'out' at work—and those who are often report experiencing a negative shift in how they are treated by colleagues when they first reveal their diagnosis.

Even when the concept of reasonable adjustments is well applied, it is limited in its capacity to conform to the neurodiversity paradigm. One issue is regarding what counts as 'reasonable'—often this judgement is made by a neurotypical person or, at the very least, is set against neurotypical norms. Universal design offers an alternative route to politicize neuronormativity at work, by rejecting the concept of adjustment—additional or different provision, against an implicit norm—and replacing it with the idea of a profoundly inclusive workplace. Universal design is not easy, and starts with fundamentals like city planning and architecture, but workplaces can make immediate steps towards it by implementing any given adjustment in as widespread a manner as possible, such as changing workplace dress codes to emphasize comfort over externally applied expectations of what is 'professional'. This is a good example of where intersectional disadvantage is also apparent—it is well known to be easier for someone who is part of a class with social power (e.g. a cisgender white man) to dress down while still being considered professional and authoritative, while someone else (e.g. a Black woman who uses a wheelchair) may be judged more harshly if she doesn't dress 'smartly'. As such, some neurodivergent people more than others will be under greater pressure to conform to narrow workplace expectations in terms of dress, hairstyle, social niceties, and so on. A universal adjustment at the national policy level which is gaining attention at the time of writing is Universal Basic Income—perhaps the single most democratizing step that a country could take towards inclusion.

Affirming complexity when it comes to employment and adult life has consequences both within a given workplace and more broadly. Another aspect of working life that serves to exclude or disadvantage neurodivergent people is the social expectations that accompany many jobs. These range from the emotional labour required of those working in the service industry to expectations around things like small talk in break spaces, after-work drinks, and colleagues' birthdays. These not only serve to exclude many neurodivergent people, but also have negative consequences for cultural diversity at work. A more specific instance of this is found in evidence that autistic people may be particularly likely to be whistle-blowers at work, detecting and reporting deviations from policy and procedure, including corruption. While this is objectively a positive contribution to the employer and industry, whistle-blowing may not be received well by colleagues and can result in autistic people being ostracized.

More broadly for society, affirming complexity involves recognizing how narrow our view of 'employment' often is—another factor which makes it hard to reliably estimate underemployment among neurodivergent people. Routinely we focus on full-time paid salaried work, and many surveys of employment fail to capture the other ways in which people may be employed in a more general sense. These include unpaid caring roles and work in the home, freelance work and self-employment, 'underground' employment such as sex work, supported employment and social enterprise, income generation through things like renting a spare room, and other kinds of gig economy working across multiple part-time jobs. Neurodivergent people may be especially drawn to these forms of employment for their increased flexibility and room for self-determination—or they may find themselves working this way due to circumstance. For example, neurodivergent adults are more likely to have neurodivergent children, some of whom may need care beyond their early years. We should resist neuronormative expectations about what constitutes a good employment outcome and work to capture all these pathways in our efforts to democratize access to fulfilling employment for neurodivergent people. A key way of organizing this will be through neurodivergent people making explicit efforts to unionize as neurodivergents, to make demands from that specific positionality.

Neurodiversity in the criminal justice system

As we noted earlier, among neurodivergent populations we often see a school-to-prison pipeline. This is similar to the levels seen among working-class Black populations, who are incarcerated in much greater numbers than those who are white and middle class. On the normalcy paradigm, the implicit assumption is that people with certain conditions or disabilities are inherently more likely to commit crime. For instance, if people with any given diagnosis are seen as deficient in empathy, or disposed to being highly impulsive, they will also be considered naturally disposed towards acting in ways that are harmful to others, more so than those who are more neurotypical. This gives the impression that there is something natural about more neurodivergent people being in prison.

Understanding the relationship between neurodivergence and the criminal justice system from a neurodiversity paradigm approach requires challenging all of this. Politicizing neuronormativity raises questions about what should count as crime in the first place. Affirming complexity requires asking whether having prisons and police are good ways to control our neurologically diverse populations.

Considering first the rates of neurodivergent people incarcerated: one study looking at a prison in Chelmsford found that over half the inmates had either dyslexia or a related learning difficulty, with similar levels found in a Texan prison. This is striking given that only around 10 per cent of the general population is dyslexic. Similarly, around one in four prisoners are reported to have ADHD, despite prevalence at only around 5 per cent of the population. High numbers are also associated with other forms of neurodivergence, from autism to schizophrenia. Thus, this seems to be a systemic issue that cuts across neurodivergent populations.

As we just noted, it has often been assumed that neurodivergent people are simply more disposed to commit crime. The neurodiversity paradigm perspective rejects this. When we say 'school-to-prison pipeline', we are already emphasizing how neurodivergent people ending up in prison stems less from individual cognitive traits and more from systemic problems that begin in school. As we have seen, neurodivergent people are routinely excluded from receiving adequate education right from their earliest years. This impacts their life chances in endless ways, including prospects for paid employment. In turn, even for those neurodivergent people who do end up in employment, as we have seen, they also face further forms of discrimination and exclusion there. All this pushes at least some neurodivergent people towards criminalized professions, such as drug dealing, sex work, and so forth.

Sometimes the way neurodivergent people comport themselves or act is seen as suspicious by members of the public and police alike. Autistic people often avoid eye contact due to sensory processing issues, but this may wrongly be viewed as a sign of dishonesty. People who hear voices and talk to themselves may be unfairly targeted due to stigmatizing representations of voice hearers and associations of 'madness' with violence. Such factors mean that in neuronormative societies, neurodivergent people are more prone to attracting police attention, despite the fact that neurodivergent people are more likely to be victims rather than perpetrators of violence. Neurodivergents are also more likely to be mistreated by the police than neurotypical people. A recent UK report found that three-quarters of those who completed suicide following police contact were neurodivergent, for instance with diagnoses of bipolar disorder or borderline personality disorder. A 2016 report from the USA indicated that the levels of mental disability among those killed by the police are up to 50 per cent. It further found that their having a mental disability was sometimes used to blame victims for being killed.

The policing and incarceration of neurodivergent people is particularly intense for those who are Black, Asian, working class, female, or nonbinary—or many of those identities. People who sit at any of these intersections are often at much greater risk. For instance, a Black autistic person experiencing sensory overload in a public space may wrongly be seen as being a threat, by both members of the public and police. Female, trans, and nonbinary neurodivergent people working in criminalized professions such as sex work (and we have already seen how this employment pathway may be more common for neurodivergent people) may also be doubly at risk of police violence, including sexual violence.

Finally, what even counts as a crime in the first place is a social rather than natural issue. Sometimes immoral things are legal while things that are not inherently problematic are criminalized. Slavery used to be legal, but clearly it should not have been. At the same time, it is far from clear that sex work should be criminalized, as this not only turns sex workers into criminals, but also makes it harder for them to access workers' rights. Once again, it is notable here that a great many neurodivergent people are either pushed towards or choose to go into sex work, and are thus at greater risk of criminalization than many neurotypicals.

Politicizing neuronormativity and affirming complexity requires recognizing that our criminal justice systems often function, in significant part, to control and incarcerate neurodivergent people who have been failed by other systems: notably employment and education. This is especially true for those who are multiply marginalized. To be clear, this is not a statement about the intentions of individual police officers, but rather about the facts of the criminal justice system as a whole. Recognizing this requires asking hard questions about whether our policing and prison systems are capable of reform or should be abolished. It may be that there are alternative ways of organizing our justice systems that would be better not just for neurodivergent people, but for everyone. Going forward, efforts should be made to centre neurodivergent perspectives in attempts to conceptualize or build these alternatives.

Applications in health and social care

Health and social care is another area in which the inequalities based in neurodiversity are both highly visible and severely consequential. Neurodivergent people require healthcare like all of us—for routine health issues, chronic conditions, at key life stages such as puberty, becoming a parent, or at the end of life, and for reasons closely connected to being neurodivergent. For example, lots of neurodivergent people will encounter healthcare providers in the context of seeking a diagnosis. Some forms of neurodivergence, like intellectual disability or autism, are associated with higher rates of health conditions such as hypermobility disorders and epilepsy—and of course the latter is itself a form of neurodivergence. Those with the highest support needs may rely on social care services across the lifespan, while others encounter them only in old age. Finally, largely due to the challenges of being neurodivergent in a society that values neuronormativity, neurodivergent people experience very high rates of mental ill-health. It is therefore imperative that health and social care systems are neurodiversity informed.

There is abundant evidence that healthcare is currently failing neurodivergent people. Stark insights come from studies on mortality, which have shown dramatically reduced life expectancy for autistic people. Recent analysis reveals that white people with a learning disability in the UK die on average at 62 years old, 18 years earlier than the general life expectancy for the UK population. Even more shocking is the fact that people with a learning disability who are from minority ethnicities are dying on average at 34 years old.

The causes of early mortality in neurodivergent people can be broadly assigned to three domains, though on the current state of the evidence it is impossible to precisely quantify their contributions. First, neurodivergent people face serious barriers to routine and acute healthcare. The precise details vary depending on the patient and their health needs, but common issues include: clinician/systemic failure to comprehend the impact of neurodiversity on symptom experiences and reporting; inaccessible modes of communication (such as telephone-only appointment booking); lack of processing time in clinical questioning and lack of familiarization time for new procedures; and failure to adapt for sensory needs. All of these phenomena make seeking help in the event of a concern, and attending routine screening appointments, a significant challenge for neurodivergent people.

A second cause of early mortality is related to specific conditions associated with neurodivergence, such as epilepsy, or cardiovascular vulnerabilities in people with Down syndrome. Not only do these conditions directly increase risk of mortality, but they compound the negative impacts of healthcare inaccessibility, because they increase the amount of healthcare support required by neurodivergent people and the severity of outcome if that care is not received. For example, during the Covid-19 pandemic, meta-analysis showed that people with intellectual disabilities were at significantly higher risk of premature mortality, and they were more at risk than any other disabled group. In the most egregious cases, neurodivergent people may be denied life-saving care because their lives are considered lower value or their quality of life is presumed to be inferior.

The third and final major cause of early mortality is suicide—as is often the case, the clearest insights come from studies with autistic people showing much higher rates of suicidal thoughts, suicide attempts, and dying by suicide. However, there is also evidence that risk of suicidality is increased for other neurodivergent people too. Moreover, suicidality has been directly related both to internalized ableism and masking of neurodivergence, suggesting that suicide risk in autistic people is not driven by genetic or neurobiological vulnerability, but by neuronormative forces that also apply to non-autistic neurodivergent people.

These neuronormative forces are also apparent when neurodivergent people access healthcare services for reasons more directly related to being neurodivergent—for example when seeking a diagnosis of ADHD or treatment for OCD. Neurodivergent people must first demonstrate that they are sufficiently different from the norm, and disabled by those differences, to quality for the affirmation that can come from a diagnosis. As we have discussed, the diagnostic process frequently serves the needs of the system more than the needs of the patient. One specific aspect of this is that giving a diagnosis is partly predicated on the need to limit access to resources, in denial of the socio-emotional value of diagnosis in a society which holds independent clinical validation in extremely high regard. If an individual is diagnosed, for example with an anxiety disorder, they are then permitted to access a post-diagnostic pathway in which support is provided. This is emphatically not necessarily the case—autistic people diagnosed as adults, for example, frequently report being provided with a few pamphlets and sent on their way. However, *if* a post-diagnostic support or treatment pathway is available, it will frequently be framed around a neuronormative agenda in which the features used to identify the best-fit diagnosis for an individual are also presumed to be in need of modification. This is a classic error in healthcare, based in the normalcy paradigm whereby anything atypical is also considered undesirable or dysfunctional. Instead, healthcare services that affirm complexity should pivot post-diagnosis, to a process of co-defining support needs and/or treatment targets with the individual. Importantly, this process will be shaped by knowledge of the diagnosis, but will not necessarily target the same behaviours used to make that diagnosis (e.g. atypical eye-contact in autism, hyperactivity in ADHD).

Social care is also a domain in which neuronormativity has a toxic effect. Neurodivergent people will frequently find themselves using social care services, with people with a learning disability in particular being some of the main long-term recipients of social care provision. In addition, of course, many neurodivergent people will find themselves living in residential social care—nursing homes—as they grow old. The danger here arises from the control the organization and its staff then have over residents. They will make decisions about every aspect of the environment and routine, and this is unlikely to take account of neurodiversity. Indeed, nursing homes for older people have been described as a form of carceral system, given the barriers to leaving these spaces once they have been entered.

One key way to affirm complexity in health and social care is to recognize and capture the expertise of neurodivergent staff more effectively. The National Health Service is one of the world's largest employers, with well over one million staff. Estimates of the collective prevalence of neurodivergence are always hard, but based on figures of 1 in 5 from UK schools, even accounting for underemployment of neurodivergent people, we would therefore expect to see many tens of thousands of neurodivergent people working in public healthcare in the UK. We should not fall into the trap of assuming that all neurodivergent people can automatically and effortlessly 'click' with each other at an individual level, nor should we deny the ability of neurotypical people to provide excellent care and support to neurodivergent folk. However, the expertise of neurodivergent practitioners in health and social care can and must be harnessed in leadership roles, quality improvement work, and pathway or service design to maximize neuroinclusion in this life-or-death context.

Chapter 4
Neurodiversity and collective liberation

So far we have covered the basic theory of neurodiversity, how this theory is applied in research, and how adopting a neurodiversity framework allows us to understand the kinds of problems neurodivergent people tend to face in modern capitalist societies. Building on this, here we consider some more general key components of the movement's political aims. While the neurodiversity movement is sometimes described as a rights movement, it is more appropriate to describe it as seeking justice and liberation for neurodivergent people by changing society in such a way that ends the neuronormative domination we have suggested is a systemic feature of the modern world. To make what we mean clear, we begin this chapter by considering the importance of human rights while also acknowledging the limitations of a rights-based approach. In particular, we suggest that rights still tend to leave the most marginalized neurodivergent people worse off than those who are more privileged. Given this shortcoming, we then turn to consider how neuronormativity is intertwined with other forms of normativity relating to race, social class, gender, and sexuality. This helps us see how neurodivergent liberation is not a single, isolated ideal, but rather an ideal that is intimately bound up with the liberation of all oppressed people everywhere.

Human rights

The disability rights movement is a global collective movement for the recognition and realization of the human rights of disabled people. All around the world, including in countries which would otherwise consider themselves upholders of international human rights legislation, the rights of disabled people are denied in ableist systems. For example, the USA social security system means that many disabled people who marry face a reduction in, or total loss of, a range of benefits including Medicaid and Medicare. Also in the USA, there are still centres where residents with a learning disability receive electric shocks aimed at modifying behaviour. This practice has been plausibly described as 'torture' by disability activist groups. In 2019, the UK—another wealthy and would-be progressive nation—was judged particularly inferior when it came to protecting disabled people from poverty. In those nations which have a poor track record on human rights, disabled people can face particular persecution. Disabled people may be subject to imprisonment, seclusion, shackling, starving, and 'treatment' via painful and unethical means.

The disability rights movement works to challenge and eradicate these practices and thereby uphold both fundamental and universal human rights (e.g. to freedom from torture), but also more disability-specific rights such as the right to reasonable adjustments at work. To the extent that neurodiversity is also a rights-based movement, it also aims to achieve the rights of neurodivergent people (who may or may not also identify as disabled). This correspondence between the disability rights movement—in many ways a 'parent' to the neurodiversity movement—and the neurodiversity movement puts paid to any suspicion that the neurodiversity movement denies disability. Importantly, fighting for the rights of neurodivergent people includes fighting for their right to clinical diagnosis, treatment, support, adjustments, accommodations, evidence-based practices, and expert guidance. Not all of these things will be relevant to every neurodivergent person at all times, but they are all part of the panoply of rights to which neurodivergent people are entitled.

However, there is a limitation to positioning the neurodiversity movement simply as the pursuit of these rights. Securing the rights listed above for all neurodivergent people does not ensure justice. In particular, a large majority of mechanisms to deliver the rights of neurodivergent people involve post-hoc modifications to systems which, at heart, fail to affirm complexity. Moreover, rights are often harder to attain for multiply marginalized neurodivergent people—who may not have support or funds to establish the implementation of their rights in practice—and thus can even help reproduce inequality as much as combat it. It is important to recall here bell hooks's notion of the 'imperialist white-supremacist capitalist patriarchy', and to recognize that rights, while necessary, will never be dispensed equally in this system. With these limitations in mind, there is reason to think we should be pursuing the kinds of fundamental socio-political and cultural shifts which mean that neurodivergent people can succeed without having first to prove the degree of need and then request a 'special' measure. This includes understanding ableism as a broader global system, but also necessitates understanding how it relates to other systems of domination.

Gender, sexuality, and neuroqueering

One area where more fundamental change might be needed is in relation to what might be called cisheteropatriarchy—the broader system of power and domination that centres men, cisgendered, and straight people while oppressing women, queer, and trans people. The relationship between neurodivergence, gender, and sexuality is complex, but there are several things worth drawing attention to in these regards.

The first thing to note is that neurodivergent people who are also members of oppressed or marginalized gender or sexuality groups tend to experience more complex forms of oppression. For instance, women with intellectual disabilities have experienced sexual abuse at much higher rates than either women without intellectual disability or men with intellectual disability. In the not-so-distant past, women with intellectual disability—especially Black women—have also often been forcibly sterilized to stop them reproducing. To give another example, autistic people who are also transgender often face intersecting forms of stigma, and their gender identity is sometimes dismissed as a 'symptom' of being autistic, or their ability to identify their own gender is questioned. These examples illustrate how gender and neurodivergence are often associated with intersecting forms of oppression that manifest in a variety of ways.

It is also worth noting here that struggles parents sometimes have with neurodivergent children are also determined partly by gendered and patriarchal norms. For instance, historically children were raised more communally, in extended families and involving other members of local communities. But various complex changes through the 19th and 20th centuries enforced the nuclear family as the core site of reproduction and care, while simultaneously enforcing most of the caring duties on mothers. This has made it harder to raise all children, but can be especially hard when those children have additional needs. Gendered parenting roles mean that the consequences fall on the shoulders of women more than on men, with consequences for their careers and personal well-being.

Moreover, culturally specific and gendered expectations about how children will behave (e.g. boys are adventurous, energetic, and bold; girls are delicate, gentle, and sweet) can lead to negative judgement on both children and their parents when those children fail to conform. Neurodivergent children may be especially likely to fail against gendered norms of behaviour and interest—girls with ADHD might be considered too active and noisy; boys with dyspraxia might struggle to fit in with activities heavily centred on team sports. Conversely, adherence to gendered expectations can act to mask neurodivergence. For example, a young woman's interests in make-up or celebrity gossip may be considered 'appropriate', and the intensity of their focus—a potential clue that they could be autistic—may be missed. A boy who avoids reading and spends his time outdoors might be thought of as having a typical male preference for rough-and-tumble, his dyslexia going undiagnosed and reading problems unaddressed. In this we see how efforts to challenge patriarchal structures and norms around motherhood and parenting may also be helpful for neurodivergent children.

Beyond such intersectional issues, intersecting power dynamics manifest not just in how neurodivergent people are treated and spotted, but also in how different forms of neurodivergence are represented or understood in the first place. For instance, autism has traditionally been represented as a mainly male diagnosis, but in recent decades female and nonbinary autistics have campaigned to gain greater recognition. What has become clearer is that traditional stereotypes of autistic people, and the diagnostic tools that enshrine them, are overly biased towards interests and behaviours socially coded as male—for instance being interested in mathematics or engineering. Not only does this reinforce outdated gendered assumptions, it also does so in a way that contributes to a lack of recognition for female and nonbinary autistic people. Another example is borderline personality disorder. This is a contested yet widely diagnosed condition associated with traits such as fear of abandonment, feelings of emptiness, unstable social relationships, and other related tendencies. Notably, it is mainly diagnosed in women and girls, including many who are queer, often when they break expected gender and sexual norms in ways that are seen as problematic by society. Neurodiversity proponents have thus often noted how the construct is used to reinforce misogynistic and heterosexual norms. However, it should also be noted that there is disagreement among neurodiversity proponents whether it should be abolished or reclaimed through a neurodiversity paradigm perspective.

When it comes to sexuality, it is worth again considering how homosexuality (to use the historical term) was pathologized as a mental disorder for much of the 20th century. From the 1960s to the 1980s especially, significant efforts were made by psychologists and psychiatrists to develop treatments or cures for same-sex attraction—efforts now known as conversion therapy. In practice, these attempts were incredibly harmful, causing mental health problems rather than healing them. In fact, homosexuality was only depathologized in the UK and USA in 1980, although even then elements of the pathologization have been retained in other diagnoses. For instance, from 1980, the diagnosis of ego dystonic homosexuality was developed and used for some years for queer people who are suffering from mental health problems relating to their sexuality. Moreover, far from being a one-off, other people who break gendered and sex norms have also often been wrongly pathologized, for instance intersex and trans people.

One way of making sense of such cases is to consider how intimately intertwined gendered and sexual norms are with neuronormativity. What is considered 'normal' in all of these regards grew together historically, while interacting in complex ways, and this is why they are hard to separate still today. For instance, autism was first pathologized, mainly in boys, in Nazi Germany. Notably this was a period where gender norms were highly restrictive and boys and men were supposed to exhibit a 'soldier mentality'. In this context, boys who were more solitary were increasingly seen as a problem to be fixed. The Nazis murdered many autistic people—not just boys, but also many girls with intellectual disability—alongside Jews, Sinti, queers, and other targets of Nazi ideology. Once we recognize how closely intertwined neuronormativity is with these other norms, we can see that neurodivergent liberation is intimately intertwined with trans and queer liberation as well as with the liberation of women from patriarchy, and that this will be good for us regardless of which gender or sexuality we have. A commitment to the neurodiversity paradigm's principle of politicizing neuronormativity thus also requires recognizing how our sexed and gendered norms are, far from being natural, the products of specific historical conditions and can often be oppressive.

One good thing that has begun to come out of this is new ways of pushing back against intersecting axes of oppression, with this activism being led by neurodivergent women, queer, and nonbinary people. One helpful concept and practice that has emerged from the recognition of this, for instance, is that of 'neuroqueering'. This describes a form of behaving—or performing—that seeks to challenge broader social norms at the point where gender norms and neuronomativity intersect. Neuroqueering is hard to define, but one way of understanding it is as committing to living in ways that playfully resist the ways in which these norms constrain all of us, to seek out new and healthier ways of living. In line with this, new forms of neurodivergent feminist and queer organizing will most likely be necessary for neurodivergent liberation in the long run.

Race, decolonization, and neuroexpansiveness

Like the relationship between neurodivergence and gender, we also see similarly complex relations and interactions when it comes to neurodiversity and race. The first thing to note here is that, historically, conceptions of normal mental functioning, intelligence, and so forth grew along with the rise of white supremacy and have remained intimately intertwined with them. As European empires colonized parts of Africa and as the field of psychiatry was beginning to emerge, for instance, psychiatrists in Britain wrote about the inferiority of African and indigenous peoples around the world, comparing non-disabled members of oppressed races to mentally disabled white Brits. European empires also brought psychiatric institutions to many colonies globally, where Black and indigenous peoples were often pathologized and treated in uniquely cruel and dehumanizing ways. As such the normalcy paradigm was not just enforced on neurodivergent people in the imperial core, but also used as a tool of colonization around the globe.

This is not just a historical problem. Today, Black and Brown neurodivergent people in white majority nations such as the UK and USA are more likely to encounter a range of issues such as police violence, discrimination, and hate crimes. Consider, for instance, how a white neurodivergent person acting in ways seen as odd in public might be seen as merely eccentric, while a Black neurodivergent person acting the same way might be seen as dangerous. In such an instance, (probably white) members of the public might call the police, and once this happens the chances of violence against the Black neurodivergent person escalate dramatically. Beyond the imperial core, writers such as Frantz Fanon have emphasized how colonialism and racism impact the mental health, and individual and collective psyches, of colonized peoples in complex and insidious ways. Thus white supremacy and colonialism are intertwined with neuronormativity in different ways in different contexts.

As with gender, our dominant representations of neurodivergence also tend to have racialized biases. For instance, autism has often been represented as not just male, but also white and middle class. This has stifled recognition and state support for Black autistics, especially those who are female or nonbinary. Further back, in the 1960s Black civil rights protesters in the United States were pathologized as having a 'protest psychosis' to dismiss their anti-racist activism. Thus, people from marginalized racial or ethnic groups can either be excluded from useful diagnoses or given harmful ones, in ways that uphold economic inequality.

Recognition of such issues has led to decolonial work by neurodivergent scholars of colour. For instance, Arya Thampuran's work examines mental health by drawing on a range of resources from across the majority world that offer alternatives to dominant biomedical framings. At the same time, it is worth considering how the neurodiversity movement needs to focus more on decolonial efforts. In a recent article, neurodiversity proponents Vishnu KK Nair, Warda Farah, and Mildred Boveda identify how the neurodiversity paradigm has retained an epistemic whiteness and focus on the Global North that needs to be overcome for the liberatory goals of the movement to be realized.

Because of how closely neuronormativity and racialized norms are intertwined, Ngozi Alston, a Black autistic writer, has proposed the term 'neuroexpansive' rather than 'neurodivergent' specifically as a term for Black people (and Black people only) to use. This emphasizes, in Alston's words, how 'neurotypical' will 'never be able to accurately describe Black bodyminds' on the grounds that Black people have never been considered neurotypical. This kind of new, historically informed theoretical work seeks to help build an analysis for autonomous Black communities seeking to resist white supremacy and colonialism from a neurologically disabled perspective. In line with this example, it seems imperative for neurodiversity advocates to recognize how closely intertwined neuronormativity and white supremacy are when understood as systemic global forces. As with gender and sexuality, liberation for neurodivergents is also intimately bound up with liberation from racial inequality and the global systems that underpin it.

Finally, it is crucial to note that the roots of the neurodiversity movement lie largely in the Global North, and much of the work contributing to arguments in this book has been generated by scholars in Europe and North America, drawing on research samples with limited racial, ethnic, and cultural diversity. Recently, neurodiversity activists have written about the global potential of the neurodiversity paradigm, while also noting that there is a danger that exporting this theoretical model unthinkingly from WEIRD (Western, Educated, Industrialized, Rich, Democratic) to non-WEIRD societies risks recapitulating the harms of colonialism. One challenge for the movement as it stands is to learn from culturally diverse ways of conceptualizing what we are calling neurodiversity and cultivate space for those to contribute to our understanding and socio-political goals. We must work collectively to uplift those of us from low- and middle-income countries and the Global South, recognizing the dangers such pioneers may face in societies which reject neurodivergence particularly powerfully. Efforts towards this can be seen in projects such as the 'Fund for Community Reparations for Autistic People of Color's Interdependence, Survival, and Empowerment', which is based in the USA but has global reach. At the same time, those of us in the Global North must be vigilant against the risk of presuming our largely Western conceptions of neurodivergence are the only or best way of achieving neurodivergent liberation.

Neurodiversity and anti-capitalism

A related question regards whether neurodivergent people can be liberated from the normalcy paradigm and oppressive norms under capitalism at all. At the moment capitalism is a global economic system that—aside from a few pockets of resistance—none of us can escape. As such, a fair amount of neurodiversity advocacy has sought to attain rights within capitalism rather than challenging that system itself. Much diversity and inclusion work, for instance, is about getting more neurodivergent people into work through recognizing neurodivergent 'strengths'. This does help some individuals, but leaves the deeper structure of capitalist society wholly intact.

However, a view from anti-capitalist neurodiversity advocates is that neuronormativity and the normalcy paradigm are products of capitalism itself and reflect the workings of this broader system in important ways. Note for instance that within capitalism each person has to compete against all others to work, and—when it comes to work—we are primarily defined by our perceived or actual potential for productivity. Within this system, our neurological and bodily norms have restricted considerably, especially following the industrial revolution and then more recent shifts towards service industry and information-based jobs that require greater emotional and attentive capacities. These shifts have meant that, instead of working as family units or with local communities, each individual is increasingly measured against everyone else in terms of their emotional and cognitive performance. Hence many job application processes now include cognitive and personality tests that do not just discriminate against neurodivergent people, but also are part of what constitutes our cultural neuronormativity.

Looked at this way, the normalcy paradigm can be seen as having arisen in part to reinforce the norms of capitalism. But if this is so, then it's not clear to what extent it will be possible to truly overcome the normalcy paradigm while we remain in this economic system. If this is convincing, then efforts to promote diversity initiatives, get more neurodivergent people into work, and reduce stigma will only have limited impact without changing the deeper economic structures of society. Thus, for proponents of anti-capitalist neurodiversity, neurodivergent liberation is intimately intertwined with the liberation of the working class from an unjust economic system. This requires neurodivergent people organizing as workers—or would-be workers—in unions, as voting blocks, or in revolutionary activism and protest to make demands on the state and ultimately to change the nature of the state in order to work towards neurodivergent—and collective—liberation.

Chapter 5
Current debates

Throughout this book we have explored the meaning and potential of the concept of neurodiversity, and the neurodiversity paradigm, to reimagine systems. The nature of the arguments and evidence presented will have made clear how early we are on the journey to neurodivergent liberation, and how much is still to be determined. In that context, we review here some key areas for open debate which have not yet been directly addressed in the preceding chapters.

Neurodiversity and learning disability

In the preceding discussions, we have often drawn attention to the specific inequalities to which people with a learning disability are vulnerable. A common accusation levelled against the concept of neurodiversity and its proponents in the neurodiversity movement is that it excludes people with a learning disability. As a reminder, we use the term 'learning disability' as it is used in the UK, to describe a specific diagnosis made when an individual has significant difficulty understanding complex information or learning new skills, often diagnosed in the presence of an IQ test score below 70. It is worth taking a moment to examine the validity of this idea and why it arises so often.

Learning disability is a naturally occurring form of neurodivergence, sometimes linked to heritable genetic variants (e.g. fragile x syndrome), sometimes arising *de novo* (e.g. Down syndrome), but often having no known biological cause. While there is no good reason for people with a learning disability to not have equal value in our society, this principle is rarely true in practice. In many Western societies, a historic value system that placed a premium on the lives of the wealthy has been seamlessly replaced by a value system based on intelligence—if not formally tested then informally judged. We have allowed ourselves to think that valuing intelligence, or some correlate of that (educational qualifications, verbal fluency, business acumen, income), is a fair system. Since intelligence is distributed equally between people of different genders, races, ethnicities, and sexualities, we can argue that a focus on intelligence can help to combat inequalities of opportunity in schools and workplaces, where attainment is both measured and highly prized. However, by definition a focus on intelligence as a value system excludes people with a learning disability, just as reliably and unacceptably as a focus on height would disadvantage women. Thus, adoption of a neurodiversity model entails a rejection of the supremacy of IQ as a marker of human worth. Until we understand and apply this manifestation of the neurodiversity paradigm, we will not be inclusive of people with a learning disability.

One reason why this mismatch—between many public accounts of the neurodiversity movement and the inclusion and liberation of people with a learning disability—might arise is because for many neurodivergent people, advocating for their rights entails highlighting their intellectual capacities. Individuals should clearly be allowed, and in fact enabled and encouraged, to understand their abilities, to develop them to their full potential, and to make these apparent to others—particularly teachers and employers. We can all draw self-esteem, joy, and opportunity from identifying the things we are good at, and doing those things. However, we need to guard against the conflation of these talents with our value as human beings. While a facility with written language might be highly valuable for a journalist, or mathematical skills may be valued in the financial services industry, such contextualized value does not apply when considering the fundamental equal value, and rights, of every member of the human race. Individual neurodivergent people have every right to advertise their talents and push back against assumptions that they lack ability, but we must collectively be careful to do this in a way that doesn't make talent or intellect a proxy for individual worth.

In order to politicize neuronormativity, neurodiversity must be understood in relation to societal and interpersonal phenomena such as stereotypes, stigma, prejudice, and discrimination. The experience of neurodivergent people is heavily dictated by these forces. This is undoubtedly specifically true for people with a learning disability, but rarely recognized as such. In particular, an unthinking adherence to the legitimacy of intelligence-as-value can justify a failure to facilitate people with a learning disability to have paid employment, opportunities for friendship, romance, and a sex life, or autonomy in a general sense. This is an example of social injustice at work, and yet is rarely perceived as such. It is true that the facilitation of autonomy may require intensive resourcing and skilled support. There will be some individuals for whom making choices will always be dependent on the close observations of others, reading and interpreting subtle signs and signals, with a degree of trial and error involved. As such, achieving the liberation of people with a learning disability is a test for the neurodiversity movement, but one which must be attempted.

The final way in which the neurodiversity movement can be seen to exclude people with a learning disability concerns leadership and advocacy. A great deal of thinking and writing about neurodiversity has come from autistic people, often those with postgraduate degrees, confident and fluent writers and speakers. All too often, their voices are pitched against neurotypical parents of people with a learning disability, as if only these two possible advocate groups exist. Autistic academic and community leader Mary Doherty calls this 'weaponized heterogeneity'—when the variability among neurodivergent people is used to negate their ability to advocate for each other. Of course, attempts to divide advocates on behalf of people with a learning disability into two groups are falsely based. First, there are many neurodivergent people who are parents or carers of people with a learning disability—these numbers are inflated beyond population averages due to genetics and the particularly common overlap of autism and learning disability. More profoundly, it is wrong to presume that there exist two separate categories of autistic people, with a clear space between on the one hand autistic people who are community leaders and activists with no learning disability, and on the other those with a learning disability who are supported in institutions—Mel Baggs's shared experience provides a powerful challenge to this crude dichotomy. And finally, many people with a learning disability can advocate for themselves, especially if provided with suitable facilitation and a platform.

What all this means is that when leaders in the neurodiversity movement campaign for change and draw attention to the inequalities that need to be broken down, it is both easy and common for others to claim that people with a learning disability are not being represented in those arguments. We contend that such claims reinforce the need for the neurodiversity movement. Application of the neurodiversity paradigm to the specific case of people with a learning disability is required to emphasize a legitimate basis for equal value, rejecting the hegemony of intellect, and to draw attention to the inequalities that mean their own perspectives are so rarely heard and their autonomy is so rarely realized.

Neurodiversity-lite

The neurodiversity movement is still relatively young and, as such,
vulnerable to misinterpretation and wilful exploitation. We refer
to the deployment of neurodiversity language, or partial adoption
of some neurodiversity concepts, without deep engagement
with the scholarship and principles of the movement, as
'neurodiversity-lite'. This name, however, belies the deeply
toxic potential of this flavour of discourse and action.

The first form of neurodiversity-lite is most commonly observed
when terminology from the movement is adopted, but overlaid on
existing practices without underlying change taking place. It is
surprisingly easy to adopt phrases like 'neurodiversity-informed'
within systems which follow the normalcy paradigm. For example,
a new clinical pathway for broad-based neurodevelopmental
assessment of adults, which provides concurrent assessment for
and diagnosis of autism and ADHD, might call itself a
neurodiversity-informed pathway, because it recognizes the
frequent co-occurrence of these two diagnostic categories. To
some degree, such a system is working to affirm complexity, but
there are many ways that same system may fail to be fully
neurodiversity affirmative. For instance, there might also be
efforts to limit the number of diagnoses given based on an
erroneous concern about there being 'too many' adults seeking a
diagnosis. Post-diagnosis, the clinical pathway might offer a
neuronormative treatment pathway, rather than challenging this
model. While this example is fictional, our point here is to note
how straightforward it is to adopt neurodiversity language in a
manner which passes superficial inspection without deeply
engaging with the tenets of the movement.

Similar cosmetic changes are possible in schools, universities,
workplaces, and social care settings. In most cases, our informal
analysis suggests that this kind of neurodiversity-lite occurs in two

scenarios. One is when progressive people, perhaps recognizing that current systems are flawed, come across the word 'neurodiversity' and attempt to apply it in the mistaken (and doubtless subconscious) belief that a combination of positive intentions and the latest terminology is equivalent to meaningful change. Such people could be open to deeper shifts in practice, but may fail to recognize that these have not occurred. The other is when organizations feel under pressure to 'move with the times', while fundamentally uncritical of their existing modes of operation. They may more consciously choose to make the minimum possible concession to the growing neurodiversity movement by relabelling systems, while actively avoiding more profound changes.

A second form of neurodiversity-lite is found when bad actors manipulate and wilfully misrepresent the ideas associated with neurodiversity, to their own selfish ends. A private practitioner might refer to their clients as 'neurodiverse' and reframe exploitative or damaging 'therapeutic' practices as neurodiversity informed, in order to make them seem more acceptable to worried parents. Worse still are cases where people reject the neurodiversity movement on the basis of false statements, such as the contention that the neurodiversity movement is not inclusive of people with a learning disability. In the most concerning scenarios neurodiversity advocates may be positioned as a powerful lobby, rather than as a marginalized minority, as a way to resist their advocacy.

Neurodiversity-lite thrives in part because of a general lack of knowledge about neurodiversity activism and scholarship. In 2023, a search on PubMed—a database for academic biomedical research—revealed just 403 results when seeking papers that use neurodiverse, neurodiversity, neurodivergent, or neurodivergence in the abstract or title. Of these, 85 per cent were published in 2021 or later. In reality, this paltry number is a massive underestimate of the wider corpus of neurodiversity scholarship, and also an unrepresentative selection. Much of the most important writing on neurodiversity is unlikely to appear in such a search, because it is published on blogs, in books, or delivered in speeches. Academics in neurodiversity-adjacent fields (e.g. developmental psychology, neuropsychiatry) searching via conventional methods will miss this work as they attempt to bring the topic into the leading outlets of the academic establishment. The result is the absence of the writing of leading thinkers in the neurodiversity movement from reference lists of influential journal articles. The alternative of citing websites or social media posts risks inadvertently reinforcing the misapprehension of neurodiversity as an unscientific, cultural trend rather than a philosophical, political, and scientific construct based in decades of thought and writing. Nonetheless, academics writing about neurodiversity and examining its applications have a responsibility to engage with the underlying scholarship on the topic.

Meanwhile, practitioners and families of neurodivergent people face different barriers to understanding, familiar when it comes to translation of all sorts of academic ideas and research findings into practice: paywalled journal articles, academic jargon, and lack of time and resources to engage with research. In this context, a range of people who play crucial roles in relation to neurodivergent people—researchers, teachers, clinicians, social workers—lack the knowledge they need to spot neurodiversity-lite and guard against it.

Why is such vigilance necessary? We contend that neurodiversity-lite is excessively damaging to the goals of the neurodiversity movement and to the lives of neurodivergent people. Superficial adoption of language actually hinders deeper change, by giving the impression that change has already taken place. Neurodivergent people using services or working in environments that claim to be neurodiversity informed (but are not) will not experience the benefits that come from affirming complexity and politicizing neuronormativity. Collectively, the false claims of critics of the movement may start to look plausible when judged against systems that have failed to engage deeply with neurodiversity. For example, organizations that claim that neurodiversity is about recognizing superpowers and celebrating special talents can reinforce the critique that the movement excludes people with a learning disability.

Another mirror-image issue is the case of organizations that are doing powerful work that treats neurodivergent ways of being as equal and valid, and destigmatizes neurodiversity-related differences, without using neurodiversity language. In this scenario, an over-focus on terminology rather than attending to core beliefs and principles can result in excellent practice being overlooked. Less mainstream approaches to education, such as Montessori or Steiner schools, may be deeply neurodiversity affirming, without ever using the language of neurodiversity. Formal structures may promote specific types of approach, making it even harder to distinguish between practices. For example, until recently Applied Behaviour Analysis was singled out for special mention in the guidelines of the American Medical Association, and this directly led to ABA—a behaviourist intervention widely seen as a form of abuse or conversion therapy by many autistic people—having a privileged status in relation to coverage under private health insurance policies. This drives autism support providers to brand what they are doing as ABA regardless of the detail of the practice, creating an ABA-monolith which disguises wide variations in specifics and ethos. Similarly in the UK, inspection of social care services virtually requires the use of Positive Behaviour Support, again driving a range of practices to be collected under that single label and masking variability in quality and underlying principles.

The reverse phenomenon occurs often in research, where there can be a worrying disconnect between performance of progressive ideals and delivery of methodological excellence. All too often, research reports are judged as neurodiversity informed simply because they use the 'correct' language, without attention paid to the rigour and quality of the methods (whether qualitative or quantitative). Meanwhile, clinical trials and systematic reviews that deploy traditional medical research methods and perhaps also terminology (intervention, patient, symptom) may be written off without a more careful exploration of the underlying assumptions and purpose of the work. It is essential to recall that critiques of the *medical model of disability* do not automatically apply to all research conducted by medics, nor to all research using clinical methods.

We call for anyone seeking to understand and adopt a neurodiversity-affirmative approach to be thoughtful in their appraisal of practices and discourse in this space. Vocabulary alone is neither an indicator of beneficence nor of harm, and an examination of the fundamental principles and beliefs that shape the activity in question is essential.

Neurodiversity and anti-psychiatry

Another common critique of the neurodiversity movement is that it is a form and continuation of the anti-psychiatry movement from the 1960s and 1970s, and that it reproduces all the same issues as this important but, in some ways, now outdated analysis. In this view, neurodiversity proponents are seen as denying that mental illness or disorder exists, in ways that may be harmful for patients who want clinical research and support.

The first thing to say here is that the term 'anti-psychiatry' is itself highly contested and is rejected by many of those to whom it is applied. But historically it was primarily used to refer to a cluster of rogue psychiatrists and social theorists who in various ways came to see psychiatry as a form of social control, and who contested this, in the mid to late 20th century. This includes people such as Thomas Szasz, the libertarian US psychiatrist who argued that mental illness is a myth; Ronald Laing, the Scottish psychiatrist who suggested that madness is produced in families and social contexts rather than merely being biological; the Canadian sociologist Erving Goffman, who argued that asylums are social institutions and psychiatric diagnoses mere 'labels'; and Franco Basaglia, the Italian anti-fascist psychiatrist who fully believed in mental illness, but saw asylums as carceral systems and worked towards developing a more humane healthcare with no locked doors in Italy.

The dominant version of anti-psychiatry in the Anglo-American world stems primarily from Szasz, and is often associated with a blanket rejection of the very concept or idea of mental illness or the various diagnoses associated with psychiatry. While this is seen as potentially liberating by some clinicians and psychiatric survivors, it is seen by many others as a dangerous and ultimately offensive denial of the reality of mental illness and disability, which if taken seriously would undermine the rights people have to treatment through either socialized medicine systems such as the NHS or through insurance claims. Critics of neurodiversity who dismiss it as a form of this kind of anti-psychiatry see it as conceptually confused and ultimately incompatible with the liberatory aims of the movement.

There are a few things to say in response to this. First, while a small number of neurodiversity proponents do hold these views, most do not. Moreover, in fact, the neurodiversity movement did not grow out of the anti-psychiatry movement at all, and rather grew out of a quite different tradition, that of the broader disabled persons' movement and the theories of disability studies covered earlier in this book. As we have seen, in this view, even in those cases where pathologization is challenged, the concept of disability is used instead, thus retaining the demand for healthcare rights and clinical support where this is needed. Moreover, most neurodiversity proponents do seem to adopt at least some conception of mental illness or disorder for at least some conditions (e.g. eating disorders) where treatment can be helpful and indeed literally life-saving. As such, it is wrong to conflate neurodiversity with the Szaszian version of the anti-psychiatry tradition, and those who do this tend to lack sufficient knowledge of the history and theoretical commitments of each movement. As we have seen, neurodiversity proponents lean towards more democratic approaches to concepts and practice rather than making blanket statements (such as that mental illness is a myth) and enforcing them from above.

That said, other thinkers associated with the anti-psychiatry movement are more compatible with the neurodiversity paradigm. Franco Basaglia had no patience for wholesale denial of mental illness and instead worked closely with his patients to help collectively build a more liberatory approach to mental healthcare that was anti-carceral in its approach. Today this system still exists in Trieste, the city where the Basaglians worked, and is widely acknowledged as providing some of the best mental health services in the world. While Basaglia was working prior to the rise of the neurodiversity movement and would most likely not have been aware of the social model of disability, we suggest that his more democratic approach—which he referred to as 'democratic psychiatry'—was broadly compatible with the commitments of the neurodiversity movement. This however is no reason to dismiss the neurodiversity approach.

Similarly, R. D. Laing also has some overlap with the neurodiversity approach. He argued for an acknowledgement that madness could sometimes lead to what he called breakthrough as well as breakdown. This did not deny the struggles or need for support of people considered mad, but sought to acknowledge that the processes of madness could manifest in different ways, and were not always or necessarily bad. While Laing was writing before the invention of the social model of disability, let alone neurodiversity theory, his work also seems more compatible with the neurodiversity approach.

One reason why the neurodiversity movement may sometimes be conflated with Szaszian anti-psychiatry is because of the depathologization agenda inherent to our position. It is worth, then, being explicit about the important role of expert clinicians in neurodivergent liberation. The 2023 case of an Australian woman with symptoms of depression who was then found to have literal worms in her brain is a stark example of how bad it could be if all mental illness was attributed to non-medical factors and wholly removed from the jurisdiction of the healthcare system. In her case, having access to doctors (rather than, say, a psychotherapist) turned out to be vital for discovering that she had a worm in her brain that was causing her psychiatric symptoms. In other, more common cases, we can see how nuanced the balance between medical intervention and disability rights can be. Worldwide, pregnant people take folic acid supplements to promote healthy development of the neural tube in the early post-conception weeks—failure to do so can result in children being born with conditions such as spina bifida. This nutritional public health intervention to prevent disability is widely accepted and crucially distinct from those efforts to prevent disabled children from being born which rest on termination of pregnancy. It provides a clear example of how preventative medical intervention can be welcomed when it rests on solid ethical foundations. Doctors, nurses, neuro-psychologists, and surgeons are all central to delivering good physical and mental health outcomes to their neurodiverse patients.

Overall, then, neurodiversity should not be equated with anti-psychiatry, and its distinct history should be recognized. Neurodiversity theory tends to avoid the now outdated views associated with some forms of anti-psychiatry, such as Szasz's view that mental illness is simply a myth, and his further proposal that all state-funded healthcare relating to mental distress should thus be abolished. At the same time, many neurodiversity proponents do share important concerns with anti-psychiatry proponents, and the movement is broadly compatible with the more radically progressive anti-psychiatrists such as Basaglia, not to mention various historic and contemporary psychiatric survivor groups committed to collective liberation more broadly. Many neurodiversity proponents also work towards alternatives to psychiatry and psychology in many instances, with the hope of undermining the disciplinary power of these fields in the long run. But critique of psychiatry and rejection of its coercive power is not the same as denying the reality of mental illness or disability.

Identity politics

Another common critique of the neurodiversity movement is that it is built on a form of identity politics that is needlessly divisive, leading to an 'us and them' narrative that could hinder organizing and collaboration in practice. As such the movement is dismissed as a distraction from real political issues such as poverty, homelessness, and so on.

Overall this is a deeply misleading and unhelpful narrative. It may be the case that there is some divisiveness associated with neurodiversity activism, but it is wrong to locate the fault of this with neurodiversity proponents. Rather, as we have detailed here, the underlying issue is that neurodivergent people are actually oppressed. As such, naming the hierarchical nature of this oppression with terms such as 'neuronormative' and 'neurodivergent' is not the genesis of this divisiveness. Rather, it is a first step towards overcoming it. And this includes overcoming things such as poverty and homelessness, which are precisely problems that disproportionately impact neurodivergent people.

That said, we do acknowledge that occasionally terms such as 'autistic' or 'neurotypical' can be used in overly essentialist ways—as if these were fixed, eternal kinds of groupings—and that this can relate to individual commitments to identities. In such cases, this may undermine efforts towards liberation, which are ultimately about building a world where many such diagnoses would no longer be needed. That said, this is certainly not an issue specific to neurodiversity advocacy. Rather, this is a much more general problem, perhaps especially in a neoliberal era, that impacts all social movements.

To those worried about overly essentialist conceptions of neurodivergent and neurotypical identity, we can direct them towards neurodiversity scholarship from Marxian and queer perspectives, which clarifies the historically contingent basis of these disabilities, and which does so in a way that avoids neuro-essentialism and the kind of limited political efforts sometimes associated with that.

Ultimately, while we think essentialist conceptions of neurodivergent or neurotypical identity are unhelpful, we support neurodiversity activism being confrontational, since this will be necessary for working towards genuine liberation. Neurodiversity politics is not supposed to leave the world as it is, but rather to change it, and this will require disruption, divisiveness, and confrontation in certain respects, whether in terms of how research is carried out to national policies, and everything in between.

The rise in self-identification

A common way experiences of neurodivergent disablement are dismissed is for critics to focus on the way diagnoses such as autism and ADHD have skyrocketed in recent decades. Such critics often focus on self-identification, which has driven part of this increase. They variously claim that only identification from a medical professional is valid, and that self-diagnosis is not reliable. They also often complain that it increasingly seems that 'everyone is neurodivergent these days', which they see as a sign of over inflation of diagnostic categories. This kind of reasoning takes a valid concern—trying to understand the rise in diagnoses—but uses it to wrongly dismiss the reality of neuronormative domination experienced by all neurodivergent people.

There are many issues with such lines of reasoning. In fact, self-identification is not obviously less reliable than medical diagnosis. After all, psychiatric diagnosis is notoriously unreliable, so the bar to match it is not very high. But beyond this, such critiques fully rely on the assumptions of the pathology paradigm, for example that when it comes to disability, the true experts are always doctors and other clinicians, or that diagnostic rates of genetically based neurodevelopmental disabilities should remain roughly stable. But as we have seen, these assumptions are precisely part of what the neurodiversity paradigm challenges. Adopting the standpoint of the neurodivergent person challenges clinical authority, and viewing disablement as relationally produced between individual and environment means we should expect rates of disability to fluctuate as our environments change. So it is unclear why neurodiversity proponents should worry about those who disagree on these grounds.

Another way of thinking about the mass increase in self-identification is viewing it as a matter of consciousness raising among populations who are increasingly disabled in a world of intensifying capitalism, falling living standards, longer work hours, and impending environmental collapse. It can also be seen as part of a mass collective project of taking power back from a paradigm that gives clinicians too much power over neurodivergent people. From this view, while there remains good reason to seek medical evaluation in certain cases (e.g. when there is a parasitic worm in your brain), and while mis-identification still remains a potential issue, the mass increase in self-identification should not be seen as a problem in itself. Rather, it is a sign that our society is disabling more and more people, and thus needs to be radically changed.

In this context it is also possible to imagine a future in which diagnostic and/or self-identification rates also decrease. Neurodivergent people self-identifying or seeking a clinical diagnosis are often trying to solve a problem in their lives. This might be fairly universally conceptualized as a mismatch between expectation and reality. Neurodivergent people regularly confound others and even themselves by failing to adhere to narrow, normative expectations of behaviour and ability. If we are successful in widening those expectations again—in creating more inclusive schools, workplaces, and communities, and in having greater patience with and understanding of each other—some of those motivations to seek a diagnosis could dissipate. Our point here is not to suggest that those seeking a diagnosis today don't really need it, or that some neurodivergent people are more 'real' than others. Rather we wish simply to acknowledge that divergence is necessarily referenced against typicality and social norms. Systems that widen our understanding of what is typical, affirming complexity and accommodating neurodiversity, may result in a lessening drive for categorization.

Co-production as a method of neurodiversity-informed change

Throughout this book we have argued for the need for change. Frequently, the requirements are radical and fundamental. For readers feeling helpless in the face of such intimidating ambitions, we advocate for the adoption of co-production—both as a mechanism of change, but also as an end, in and of itself. Co-production here is used as an umbrella term referring to a range of ways of working together, across traditional boundaries. This could mean neurodiverse teams of people in any setting; academics working with partners outside the ivory tower; clinicians partnering with patients; or teachers collaborating with pupils and parents.

Co-production offers a number of immediate advantages in line with the principles of the neurodiversity movement. Bringing different perspectives together honours the requirement to affirm complexity. Diverse teams working together harness the key strength inherent in neurodiversity—the fact that we bring different experiences to the table. In doing so, we each challenge our worldview, expand our understanding, and increase our empathy. At a functional level, diverse teams have greater potential to anticipate challenges and identify solutions to them. Co-production also holds potential for emancipation of those involved, in particular when less powerful cohorts gain new skills through their co-working, and adopt leadership roles in the process.

Longer term, co-production must be central to our plans to democratize systems. Simply put, we cannot entrust neurodivergent liberation to one group, however well educated or thoughtful they may be. Transfer of power from one group to another is no guarantee of benign results, as starkly illustrated in Orwell's *Animal Farm*. By working together we can continue to learn from each other, checking and balancing as we go, distributing rather than merely transferring power.

The neurodiversity movement and its ongoing attempt at a paradigm shift has great liberatory capacity, and should be understood as part of a broader intersectional struggle for liberation. In this, it has particular potential to revolutionize research and practice. In turn, this should impact how we organize society more generally, from education, through the workplace, to criminal justice, healthcare, and beyond. As an ideal the neurodiversity paradigm is worth fighting for.

Yet at the same time, it remains far from clear that this potential will be realized. To do so will take great collective effort and organization, across borders and in tandem and solidarity with other movements, over many decades. It requires great sacrifice from many and needs a vast change in the power structures that govern neuronormativity.

Without this mass, collective effort, it seems likely that neurodiversity-lite will become the dominant variant of the approach. This may help some people in particular ways, but will ultimately just reform the normalcy paradigm rather than bringing a revolution towards the neurodiversity paradigm. For those who see the neurodiversity paradigm as worth fighting for, it will be up to each and all of us to work towards not just neurodiversity affirmation, but also collective liberation.

References and further reading

Preface

Cheng, Y., Tekola, B., Balasubramanian, A., Crane, L., & Leadbitter, K. (2023). Neurodiversity and community-led rights-based movements: Barriers and opportunities for global research partnerships. *Autism, 27*(3), 573–7.

Crenshaw, K. (1991). Mapping the margins: Intersectionality, identity politics, and violence against women of color. *Stanford Law Review, 43*(6), 1241–99.

'imperialist white-supremacist capitalist patriarchy', p. 17 in b. hooks (2004), *The Will to Change: Men, Masculinity, and Love.* New York: Atria Books.

Nair, V. K., Farah, W., & Boveda, M. (2024). Is neurodiversity a Global Northern White paradigm? *Autism,* 13623613241280835.

Walker, N. (2021). *Neuroqueer Heresies: Notes on the Neurodiversity Paradigm, Autistic Empowerment, and Postnormal Possibilities.* Fort Worth, TX: Autonomous Press.

Chapter 1: Introducing neurodiversity

'autism-specific deception impairment' in S. Baron-Cohen (1992), Out of sight or out of mind? Another look at deception in autism. *Journal of Child Psychology and Psychiatry,* 33: 1141–55. <https://doi.org/10.1111/j.1469-7610.1992.tb00934.x>

Blume, H. (1997). Autistics, freed from face-to-face encounters, are communicating in cyberspace. *New York Times,* 30 June, downloaded on 22/09/2023 from <https://www.nytimes.com/1997/06/30/business/autistics-freed-from-face-to-face-encounters-are-communicating-in-cyberspace.html>.

Blume, H. (1998). Neurodiversity: On the neurological underpinnings of geekdom. *The Atlantic*, September issue, downloaded on 22/09/2023 from <https://www.theatlantic.com/magazine/archive/1998/09/neurodiversity/305909/>.

Botha, M., Chapman, R., Giwa Onaiwu, M., Kapp, S. K., Stannard Ashley, A., & Walker, N. (2024). The neurodiversity concept was developed collectively: An overdue correction on the origins of neurodiversity theory. *Autism*, *28*(6), 1591–4.

Crenshaw, K., Gotanda, N., Peller, G., & Thomas, K. (eds). (1995). *Critical Race Theory: The Key Writings that Formed the Movement*. New York: The New Press.

Kapp, S. (2020). *Autistic Community and the Neurodiversity Movement: Stories from the Frontline*. London: Palgrave Macmillan.

Lewis, A. C., Molina, S. J., Appelbaum, P. S., Dauda, B., Di Rienzo, A., Fuentes, A., Fullerton, S. M., Garrison, N. A., Ghosh, N., Hammonds, E. M., Jones, D. S., Kenny, E. E., Kraft, P., Lee, S. S.-J., Mauro, M., Novembre, J., Panofsky, A., Sohail, M., Neale, B. M., & Allen, D. S. (2022). Getting genetic ancestry right for science and society. *Science*, *376*(6590), 250–2.

Macmillan, M. (2000). Restoring Phineas Gage: A 150th retrospective. *Journal of the History of the Neurosciences*, *9*(1), 46–66.

Roberts, G., Quach, J., Spencer-Smith, M., Anderson, P. J., Gathercole, S., Gold, L., Sia, K.-L., Mensah, F., Rickards, F., Ainley, J., & Wake, M. (2016). Academic outcomes 2 years after working memory training for children with low working memory: A randomized clinical trial. *JAMA pediatrics*, *170*(5), e154568–e154568.

Robinson, C. J. (2021). *Black Marxism: The Making of the Black Radical Tradition*. London: Penguin Modern Classics.

Singer, J. (1999). Why can't you be normal for once in your life? From a problem with no name to the emergence of a new category of difference. In M. Corker and S. French (eds), *Disability Discourse*, 59–70. Buckingham: Open University Press.

Zentall, S., Kuester, D., & Craig, B. (2011). Social behavior in cooperative groups: Students at risk for ADHD and their peers. *Journal of Educational Research*, 104, 28–41.

'may not become fully manifest until social demands exceed limited capacities, or may be masked by learned strategies in later life' in American Psychiatric Association (2013). *Diagnostic and Statistical Manual of Mental Disorders*, 5th edn. Arlington: American Psychiatric Association.

Astle, D. E., Holmes, J., Kievit, R., & Gathercole, S. E. (2022). Annual Research Review: The transdiagnostic revolution in neurodevelopmental disorders. *Journal of Child Psychology and Psychiatry*, *63*(4), 397–417.

Bergenmar, J., Creechan, L., & Stenning, A. (2024). *Critical Neurodiversity Studies: Divergent Textualities in Literature and Culture*. London: Bloomsbury.

Botha, M., & Frost, D. M. (2020). Extending the minority stress model to understand mental health problems experienced by the autistic population. *Society and Mental Health*, *10*(1), 20–34.

Creechan, L. (forthcoming). Reading, writing, and idiocy: Sensation novels and the threat of the neurodivergent reader. *Literature and Medicine*.

Crompton, C. J., Hallett, S., Ropar, D., Flynn, E., & Fletcher-Watson, S. (2020a). 'I never realised everybody felt as happy as I do when I am around autistic people': A thematic analysis of autistic adults' relationships with autistic and neurotypical friends and family. *Autism*, *24*(6), 1438–48.

Crompton, C. J., Ropar, D., Evans-Williams, C. V., Flynn, E. G., & Fletcher-Watson, S. (2020b). Autistic peer-to-peer information transfer is highly effective. *Autism*, *24*(7), 1704–12.

Crompton, C. J., Sharp, M., Axbey, H., Fletcher-Watson, S., Flynn, E. G., & Ropar, D. (2020c). Neurotype-matching, but not being autistic, influences self and observer ratings of interpersonal rapport. *Frontiers in Psychology*, *11*, 2961.

Fletcher-Watson, S., & Bird, G. (2020). Autism and empathy: What are the real links? *Autism*, *24*(1), 3–6.

Folkerth, W. (2021). Reading Shakespeare after neurodiversity. In Leslie C. Dunn (ed.), *Performing Disability in Early Modern English Drama*, 141–57. London: Palgrave.

Forbes, M. K., Neo, B., Nezami, O. M., Fried, E. I., Faure, K., Michelsen, B., Twose, M., & Dras, M. (2023, 21 March). Elemental psychopathology: Distilling constituent symptoms and patterns of repetition in the diagnostic criteria of the DSM-5. *Open Science Framework, preprint*; <https://doi.org/10.1017/ S0033291723002544>.

Haller, B., & Preston, J. (2016). Confirming normalcy: 'Inspiration porn' and the construction of the disabled subject. In K. Ellis and M. Kent (eds), *Disability and Social Media*, 63–78. London: Routledge.

Johnson, M. L. (2021). 'Neuroqueer feminism: Turning with tenderness towards borderline personality disorder'. *Signs, 46*(3), 635–62.

Kapp, S., & Ne'eman, A. (2012). *ASD in DSM-5: What the Research Shows and Recommendations for Change.* Autistic Self-Advocacy Network, Policy Brief. <https://autisticadvocacy.org/wp-content/ uploads/2012/06/ASAN_DSM-5_2_final.pdf>.

Mardiros, M. (1989). Conception of childhood disability among Mexican-American parents. *Medical Anthropology, 12*(1), 55–68.

Milton, D., Gurbuz, E., & López, B. (2022). The 'double empathy problem': Ten years on. *Autism, 26*(8), 1901–3.

Milton, D. E. (2012). On the ontological status of autism: The 'double empathy problem'. *Disability & Society, 27*(6), 883–7.

Murray, F. (2021). *Weird Pride Day.* <https://oolong.medium.com/ weird-pride-day-232465b67dd9>.

Oliver, D. (2019). *Awkwoods: Daniel Oliver's Dyspraxic Adventures in Participatory Performance.* London: Live Art Development Agency.

Rodas, J. M. (2018). *Autistic Disturbances: Theorizing Autism Poetics from the DSM to Robinson Crusoe.* Ann Arbor: University of Michigan Press.

Sasson, N. J., Faso, D. J., Nugent, J., Lovell, S., Kennedy, D. P., & Grossman, R. B. (2017). Neurotypical peers are less willing to interact with those with autism based on thin slice judgments. *Scientific Reports, 7*(1), 1–10.

Savarese, R. J. (2018). *See It Feelingly: Classic Novels, Autistic Readers, and the Schooling of a No-Good English Professor.* Durham, NC: Duke University Press.

Sheppard, E., Pillai, D., Wong, G. T. L., Ropar, D., & Mitchell, P. (2016). How easy is it to read the minds of people with autism spectrum disorder? *Journal of Autism and Developmental Disorders, 46*, 1247–54.

ADHD Foundation (2022). *ADHD in the Criminal Justice System: A Case for Change*. Downloaded from <https://www.adhdfoundation.org.uk>.

Biederman, J., & Faraone, S. V. (2006). The effects of attention-deficit/hyperactivity disorder on employment and household income. *Medscape General Medicine, 8*(3), 12.

Cassidy, S., Bradley, L., Shaw, R., & Baron-Cohen, S. (2018). Risk markers for suicidality in autistic adults. *Molecular Autism, 9*, 1–14.

Cassidy, S., & Rodgers, J. (2017). Understanding and prevention of suicide in autism. *The Lancet Psychiatry, 4*(6), e11.

Chapman, R. (2023). *Empire of Normality: Neurodiversity and Capitalism*. London: Pluto Press.

'While the rate increased steadily…': Chen, J. L., Leader, G., Sung, C., & Leahy, M. (2015). Trends in employment for individuals with autism spectrum disorder: A review of the research literature. *Review Journal of Autism and Developmental Disorders, 2*, 115–27, at p. 117.

Freire, P. (1970). *Pedagogy of the Oppressed*. New York: Continuum Press.

Hewitt-Main, J. (2012). *Dyslexia Behind Bars*. Benfleet: Mentoring 4 U. Downloaded from <http://www.lexion.co.uk/references.html>.

Independent Office for Police Conduct. (2023). *Deaths During or Following Police Contact Statistics for England and Wales 2022/23*. Downloaded from <https://www.policeconduct.gov.uk/publications/annual-deaths-during-or-following-police-contact-report-202223>.

Koncul, A., Kelly, C., Aubrecht, K., & Bartlett, R. (2023). Long-term care homes: Carceral spaces in times of crisis or perpetually? *Space and Culture*, 26(3), 309–322. <https://doi.org/10.1177/12063312231159219>.

Kuper, H., & Smythe, T. (2023). *Are People with Disabilities at Higher Risk of COVID-19-Related Mortality? A Systematic Review and Meta-Analysis* <http://dx.doi.org/10.2139/ssrn.4356773>.

Lorde, A.. (2018). *The Master's Tools Will Never Dismantle the Master's House*. London: Penguin Classics.

Maciver, D., Rutherford, M., Arakelyan, S., Kramer, J. M., Richmond, J., Todorova, L., . . . & Forsyth, K. (2019). Participation of children with disabilities in school: A realist systematic review of psychosocial and environmental factors. *Plos One, 14*(1), e0210511.

Melling, K., Beyer, S., & Kilsby, M. (2011). Supported employment for people with learning disabilities in the UK: The last 15 years. *Tizard Learning Disability Review, 16*(2), 23–32.

Moody, K. C., Holzer III, C. E., Roman, M. J., Paulsen, K. A., Freeman, D. H., Haynes, M., & James, T. N. (2000). Prevalence of dyslexia among Texas prison inmates. *Texas Medicine, 96*(6), 69–75.

Paget, A., Parker, C., Heron, J., Logan, S., Henley, W., Emond, A., & Ford, T. (2018). Which children and young people are excluded from school? Findings from a large British birth cohort study, the Avon Longitudinal Study of Parents and Children (ALSPAC). *Child: Care, Health and Development, 44*(2), 285–96.

Perry, D. M., & Carter-Long, L. (2017). The Ruderman white paper on media coverage of law enforcement use of force and disability: A media study (2013–2015) and overview. Downloaded from <https://rudermanfoundation.org/advocacy-media/white-papers/>.

Pryke-Hobbes, A., Davies, J., Heasman, B., Livesey, A., Walker, A., Pellicano, E., & Remington, A. (2023). The workplace masking experiences of autistic, non-autistic neurodivergent and neurotypical adults in the UK. *Plos One, 18*(9), e0290001.

Race and Health Observatory. (2023). *We deserve better: Ethnic minorities with a learning disability and access to healthcare.* Downloaded from <https://www.nhsrho.org/publications/>.

Shaw, S. C., Fossi, A., Carravallah, L. A., Rabenstein, K., Ross, W., & Doherty, M. (2023). The experiences of autistic doctors: A cross-sectional study. *Frontiers in Psychiatry, 14*, 1160994.

Weinreich, L., Haberstroh, S., Schulte-Körne, G., & Moll, K. (2023). The relationship between bullying, learning disorders and psychiatric comorbidity. *BMC Psychiatry, 23*(1), 116.

Chapter 4: Neurodiversity and collective liberation

'imperialist white-supremacist, capitalist patriarchy' in bell hooks (2000), *Feminism is for Everybody: Passionate Politics.* Cambridge, MA: South End Press, p. 46.

'neurotypical' will 'never be able to accurately describe Black bodyminds' in N. Alston (2022). *Neuroexpansive™ Thoughts.*

<https://medium.com/@ngwagwa/neuroexpansive-thoughts-9db1e566d361>.

Cheng, Y., Tekola, B., Balasubramanian, A., Crane, L., & Leadbitter, K. (2023). Neurodiversity and community-led rights-based movements: Barriers and opportunities for global research partnerships. *Autism, 27*(3), 573–7.

Fanon, F. (1968). *The Wretched of the Earth*. New York: Grove Press.

Johnson, M. L. (2021). Neuroqueer feminism: Turning with tenderness toward borderline personality disorder. *Signs, 46*(3), 635–62.

Thampuran, A. (2022). *Decolonial Approaches to Reading Distress, Healing, and (Well)being in Contemporary African Diasporic Contexts*. Doctoral thesis, Durham University.

'neuroqueering' in M. Yergeau (2018). *Authoring Autism: On Rhetoric and Neurological Queerness*. Durham, NC: Duke University Press.

Chapter 5: Current debates

Baggs, M. (2019). Losing. In S. K. Kapp (ed.), *Autistic Community and the Neurodiversity Movement: Stories from the Frontline*, 77–86. Singapore: Springer Singapore.

Baron-Cohen, S. (2017). Editorial perspective: Neurodiversity—a revolutionary concept for autism and psychiatry. *Journal of Child Psychology and Psychiatry, 58*(6), 744–7.

Botha, M., Chapman, R., Giwa Onaiwu, M., Kapp, S. K., Stannard Ashley, A., & Walker, N. (2024). The neurodiversity concept was developed collectively: An overdue correction on the origins of neurodiversity theory. *Autism, 28*(6), 1591–4.

Chapman, R. (2020). The reality of autism: On the metaphysics of disorder and diversity. *Philosophical Psychology, 33*(6), 799–819.

'weaponized heterogeneity' in M. Doherty (2023). *Weaponized Heterogeneity Only Harms the Most Vulnerable Autistic People*. Spectrum, <https://doi.org/10.53053/WDPZ6657>.

Sonuga-Barke, E., & Thapar, A. (2021). The neurodiversity concept: Is it helpful for clinicians and scientists? *The Lancet Psychiatry, 8*(7), 559–61.

Walker, N. (2021). *Neuroqueer Heresies: Notes on the Neurodiversity Paradigm, Autistic Empowerment, and Postnormal Possibilities*. Fort Worth, TX: Autonomous Press.

Index

For the benefit of digital users, indexed terms that span two pages (e.g., 52–53) may, on occasion, appear on only one of those pages.

AUTISM
A Very Short Introduction
Uta Frith

This *Very Short Introduction* offers a clear statement on what is currently known about autism and Asperger syndrome. Explaining the vast array of different conditions that hide behind these two labels, and looking at symptoms from the full spectrum of autistic disorders, it explores the possible causes for the apparent rise in autism and also evaluates the links with neuroscience, psychology, brain development, genetics, and environmental causes including MMR and Thimerosal. This short, authoritative, and accessible book also explores the psychology behind social impairment and savantism and sheds light on what it is like to live inside the mind of the sufferer.

www.oup.com/vsi

CIRCADIAN RHYTHMS

A Very Short Introduction

Russell Foster

The earth's daily rotation affects just about every living creature. However, these changes are regular, rhythmic and, therefore, predictable. This near-24 hour circadian rhythm is innate: a genetically programmed clock that ticks of its own accord.

This *Very Short Introduction* explains how organisms can 'know' the time and reveals what we now understand of the nature and operation of chronobiological processes. Covering variables such as light, the metabolism, human health, and the seasons, Foster and Kreitzman illustrate how jet lag and shift work can impact on human well-being, and consider circadian rhythms alongside a wide range of disorders, from schizophrenia to obesity.

www.oup.com/vsi

COGNITIVE NEUROSCIENCE

A Very Short Introduction
Richard Passingham

Up to the 1960s, psychology regarded what happened within the mind as scientifically unapproachable. As medical research evolved, outlines of brain components and processes began to take shape, and by the end of the 1970s, a new science, cognitive neuroscience, was born.

In this *Very Short Introduction*, distinguished cognitive neuroscientist Richard Passingham gives a provocative and exciting account of the nature and scope of this relatively new field. He explains what brain imaging shows, pointing out common misconceptions, and gives a brief overview of the different aspects of human cognition: perceiving, attending, remembering, reasoning, deciding, and acting. He also considers the exciting advances that may lie ahead.

www.oup.com/vsi

CONSCIENCE
A Very Short Introduction
Paul Strohm

In the West conscience has been relied upon for two thousand years as a judgement that distinguishes right from wrong. It has effortlessly moved through every period division and timeline between the ancient, medieval, and modern. The Romans identified it, the early Christians appropriated it, and Reformation Protestants and loyal Catholics relied upon its advice and admonition. Today it is embraced with equal conviction by non-religious and religious alike. Considering its deep historical roots and exploring what it has meant to successive generations, Paul Strohm highlights why this particularly European concept deserves its reputation as 'one of the prouder Western contributions to human rights and human dignity throughout the world.

DEPRESSION
A Very Short Introduction
Jan Scott and Mary Jane Tacchi

What is depression? What is bipolar disorder? How are they diagnosed and how are they treated?

In this *Very Short Introduction*, Jan Scott and Mary Jane Tacchi give an informative account of the changing understandings of depression, manic depression and bipolar disorder, and the new treatments available to people suffering from depression—from antidepressants to mood stabilizers. They explore the association between mood disorders and physical illness, as well as the link between creativity and depression in modern-day society. Scott and Tacchi also consider what may lie ahead for those living with depression.

DREAMING
A Very Short Introduction

J. Allan Hobson

What is dreaming and what causes it? Why are dreams so strange and often hard to remember?

In this *Very Short Introduction*, J. Allan Hobson provides a new and increasingly complete picture of how dreaming is created by the brain. Hobson offers possible answers to long-held questions on activation, function, and the interpretation of dreams, and reveals how dreaming maintains and develops the mind. As well as investigating the relationship between dreaming, learning, memory, and consciousness, Hobson investigates his own dreams to illustrate and explain some of the fascinating discoveries of modern sleep science.

www.oup.com/vsi

EXISTENTIALISM
A Very Short Introduction
Thomas Flynn

Existentialism was one of the leading philosophical movements of the twentieth century. Focusing on its seven leading figures, Sartre, Nietzsche, Heidegger, Kierkegaard, de Beauvoir, Merleau-Ponty and Camus, this *Very Short Introduction* provides a clear account of the key themes of the movement which emphasized individuality, free will, and personal responsibility in the modern world. Drawing in the movement's varied relationships with the arts, humanism, and politics, this book clarifies the philosophy and original meaning of 'existentialism' - which has tended to be obscured by misappropriation. Placing it in its historical context, Thomas Flynn also highlights how existentialism is still relevant to us today.

www.oup.com/vsi

GENIUS
A Very Short Introduction
Andrew Robinson

Genius is highly individual and unique, of course, yet it shares
a compelling, inevitable quality for professionals and the general
public alike. Darwin's ideas are still required reading for every
working biologist; they continue to generate fresh thinking
and experiments around the world. So do Einstein's theories
among physicists. Shakespeare's plays and Mozart's melodies
and harmonies continue to move people in languages and
cultures far removed from their native England and Austria.
Contemporary 'geniuses' may come and go, but the idea of
genius will not let go of us. Genius is the name we give to a quality
of work that transcends fashion, celebrity, fame, and reputation:
the opposite of a period piece. Somehow, genius abolishes
both the time and the place of its origin.

www.oup.com/vsi

KNOWLEDGE
A Very Short Introduction
Jennifer Nagel

What is knowledge? Is it the same as opinion or truth? Do you need to be able to justify a claim in order to count as knowing it?

Questions like these are ancient ones, and the branch of philosophy dedicated to answering them—epistemology—has been active for thousands of years.

In this thought provoking *Very Short Introduction*, Jennifer Nagel considers the central problems and paradoxes in the theory of knowledge whilst drawing attention to the ways in which philosophers and theorists have responded to them. She incorporates methods from logic, linguistics, and psychology, and uses a number of everyday examples to demonstrate the key issues and debates.

www.oup.com/vsi

PUBLIC HEALTH
A Very Short Introduction
Virginia Berridge

Public health is a term much used in the media, by health
professionals, and by activists. But what do we mean when we
speak about 'public health'?

In this *Very Short Introduction* Virginia Berridge explores the areas
which fall under the remit of public health, and explains how the
individual histories of different countries have come to cause
great differences in the perception of the role and responsibilities
of public health organisations. Drawing on a wide range of
international examples, Berridge demonstrates the central role
of history to understanding the amorphous nature of public health
today.

www.oup.com/vsi

SEXUALITY
A Very Short Introduction
Veronique Mottier

What shapes our sexuality? Is it a product of our genes, or of
society, culture, and politics? How have concepts of sexuality
and sexual norms changed over time? How have feminist
theories, religion, and HIV/AIDS affected our attitudes to sex?
Focusing on the social, political, and psychological aspects of
sexuality, this *Very Short Introduction* examines these
questions and many more, exploring what shapes our sexuality,
and how our attitudes to sex have in turn shaped the wider world.
Revealing how our assumptions about what is 'normal' in
sexuality have, in reality, varied widely across time and place,
this book tackles the major topics and controversies that still
confront us when issues of sex and sexuality are discussed:
from sex education, HIV/AIDS, and eugenics, to religious
doctrine, gay rights, and feminism.

www.oup.com/vsi

Logic
A Very Short Introduction
Graham Priest

Logic is often perceived as an esoteric subject, having little
to do with the rest of philosophy, and even less to do with real life.
In this lively and accessible introduction, Graham Priest shows
how wrong this conception is. He explores the philosophical
roots of the subject, explaining how modern formal logic deals
with issues ranging from the existence of God and the reality
of time to paradoxes of self-reference, change, and probability.
Along the way, the book explains the basic ideas of formal
logic in simple, non-technical terms, as well as the philosophical
pressures to which these have responded. This is a book for
anyone who has ever been puzzled by a piece of reasoning.

'a delightful and engaging introduction to the basic concepts of
logic. Whilst not shirking the problems, Priest always manages to
keep his discussion accessible and instructive.'

Adrian Moore, St Hugh's College, Oxford

'an excellent way to whet the appetite for logic. . . . Even if you read
no other book on modern logic but this one, you will come away
with a deeper and broader grasp of the *raison d'être* for logic.'

Chris Mortensen, University of Adelaide

www.oup.com/vsi

LANGUAGES
A Very Short Introduction
Stephen Anderson

How many languages are there? What differentiates one language from another? Are new languages still being discovered? Why are so many languages disappearing?

The diversity of languages today is varied, but it is steadily declining. In this *Very Short Introduction*, Stephen Anderson answers the above questions by looking at the science behind languages. Considering a wide range of different languages and linguistic examples, he demonstrates how languages are not uniformly distributed around the world; just as some places are more diverse than others in terms of plants and animal species, the same goes for the distribution of languages.

Exploring the basis for linguistic classification and raising questions about how we identify a language, as well as considering signed languages as well as spoken, Anderson examines the wider social issues of losing languages, and their impact in terms of the endangerment of cultures and peoples.